DOORFRAME PULL-UP BAR WORKOUTS

Full-Body Strength Training for Arms, Chest, Shoulders, Back, Core, Glutes and Legs

Ryan George

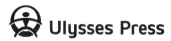 Ulysses Press

Published in the United States by
ULYSSES PRESS
P.O. Box 3440
Berkeley, CA 94703
www.ulyssespress.com

ISBN: 978-1-61243-356-1
Library of Congress Control Number 2014932304

Printed in the United States by Bang Printing

10 9 8 7 6 5 4 3 2 1

Acquisitions: Keith Riegert
Managing editor: Claire Chun
Editor: Lily Chou
Proofreader: Lauren Harrison
Indexer: Sayre Van Young
Front cover and interior design: what!design @ whatweb.com
Cover photographs: man © Rapt Productions; brick wall © Tupungato/shutterstock.com; stone background in doorframe © HolyCrazyLazy/shutterstock.com
Interior photographs: © Rapt Productions except on page 8 © Photobank gallery/shutterstock.com
Models: Tyler Eisner, Ryan George, Nadia Velasquez

Distributed by Publishers Group West

PLEASE NOTE: This book has been written and published strictly for informational purposes, and in no way should be used as a substitute for consultation with health care professionals. You should not consider educational material herein to be the practice of medicine or to replace consultation with a physician or other medical practitioner. The author and publisher are providing you with information in this work so that you can have the knowledge and can choose, at your own risk, to act on that knowledge. The author and publisher also urge all readers to be aware of their health status and to consult health care professionals before beginning any health program.

This book is independently authored and published. No sponsorship or endorsement of this book by, and no affiliation with any doorframe pull-up bar, including Iron Gym (Ontel Products Corporation), or any other trademarked brands or products mentioned or pictured, is claimed or suggested. All trademarks that appear in this book belong to their respective owners and are used here for informational purposes only. The author and publisher encourage readers to patronize the quality brands and other products mentioned and pictured in this book.

CONTENTS

PART I: OVERVIEW 1

Introduction................................. 2
About This Book.......................... 4
The Doorframe Pull-Up Bar.......... 5
The Muscles................................ 8
Components of a Movement 11
What Is Fitness?........................... 14
Keys to Success........................... 20
Nutrition and Eating Strategies............ 25
Before You Begin 29

PART II: PROGRAMS 31

How to Use This Book.................. 32
Fitness Assessments 33
Goal Setting 40
Program Design........................... 42
Templates 46
Programs 50

PART III: EXERCISES............ 93

Pull-Ups 94

Chin-Up 96
Parallel Grip Pull-Up 97
Standard Pull-Up.......................... 98
Alternate-Grip Pull-Up 99
Close-Grip Pull-Up 100
Wide-Grip Pull-Up........................ 101
Side-Facing Pull-Up...................... 102
Side-to-Side Pull-Up..................... 103
L-Shaped Pull-Up 104
Pull-Up with Leg Curl 105
Hanging Biceps Curl...................... 106

Isometric Hold (Side to Side)................ 107
Pull-Up with Press-Out 108
Pull-Up with High Leg Raise 109
Squat Thrust into Pull-Up.................. 110

Building Up to Pull-Ups 111

Scapular Pull-Up 111
Isometric Hold 112
Pull-Up with Negative Focus................ 113
Modified Pull-Up 114
Partner-Assisted Pull-Up 115
Short-Range Pull-Up (Lower Half) 116
Short-Range Pull-Up (Upper Half)........ 117
Chair-Assisted Pull-Up 118
Band-Assisted Pull-Up 119
Jumping Pull-Up 120
Jumping Pull-Up (Feet on Floor) 121

Hanging Abdominal Exercises.... 122

Hanging Leg Curl.............................. 123
Straight-Leg Raise............................. 124
Hanging Leg Curl with Rotation 125
Straight-Leg Raise Side to Side 126
Alternate Single-Leg Raise 127
Alternate Single-Leg Raise
Side to Side..................................... 128
Oblique Twist................................... 129
Half Circle....................................... 130
Full Circle.. 132
Leg Curl with Extension...................... 133
Hanging Oblique Crunch 134
Hanging Bicycle................................. 135
High Twist.. 136

■ **Push-Up-Based Exercises**............ 137

Push-Up 139

Wide Push-Up 140

Diamond Push-Up 141

Triceps Push-Up 141

Staggered Push-Up 142

Power Push-Up 143

Push-Up with Rotation 144

Total-Body Explosive Push-Up.......... 145

■ **Lower-Body Exercises** 146

Squat 146

Split Squat 147

Forward Lunge 148

Reverse Lunge................................ 149

Bridge 150

Single-Leg Bridge.......................... 151

Single-Leg Squat............................ 152

■ **Upper-Body Exercises** 153

Chair Dip....................................... 153

Floor Dip 154

Press-Up 155

Plank Walk-Up............................... 156

Standing Walk-Out.......................... 157

Handstand Shoulder Press 158

■ **Plank-Based Exercises**................. 159

Plank 161

Plank with Arm Extension 162

Side Plank 163

Plank to Side Plank 164

■ **Abdominal Exercises**.................... 165

Crunch 165

Bicycle Crunch 166

Kick-Up... 167

Leg Curl.. 168

Total-Body Crunch.......................... 168

■ **Doorframe Pull-Up Bar Floor Exercises** 169

Push-Up with Bar 169

Dip with Bar.................................. 170

Press-Up with Bar 171

Core Walk-Out 172

Frame-Assisted Sit-Up 173

Calf Raise 174

Leg Extension................................ 174

Alternate-Grip Push-Up with Bar 175

Pike Press 175

■ **Cardio-Conditioning Exercises**..... 176

Speed Squat.................................. 176

Skater 178

Shoulder Touch 179

Mountain Climber 179

High Knees.................................... 180

Squat Jump 181

Jumping Lunge............................... 182

Squat Thrust.................................. 183

■ **APPENDIX**..........................**184**

Warming Up................................... 185

Cardio... 188

Stretching & Cooling Down.............. 189

Index 193

Acknowledgments 196

About the Author 196

PART I
OVERVIEW

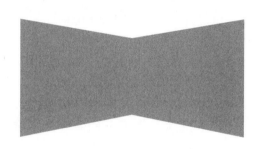

INTRODUCTION

At its core, exercise is really simple. It involves the application of a few basic but well-tested principles in order to achieve a desired result: consistency, specificity, efficiency, progression and recovery. These core principles are both easy to understand and easy to apply to any situation.

Over time and for a variety of reasons, this simplicity has become overly complicated. We're bombarded with new equipment, fad diets and trendy workouts that often make promises that are far too good to be true. While some have merit, more often than not they're simply a cash grab. Magazines have to sell issues, websites have to generate hits. As a result, we find a market oversaturated with information that's often contradictory. The problem is that, with so much misinformation flooding the market, the average person can be overwhelmed and unsure of how to proceed with an exercise program. This leads to months and years of guesswork and a process of trial and error that can be frustrating and discouraging and ultimately lead to failure.

The purpose of *Doorframe Pull-Up Bar Workouts* is to peel back the layers of misinformation in order to reveal exercise's simple roots. A second purpose is to make exercise and fitness accessible to anybody in any setting. To achieve this, I'm centering the workouts around one of the absolute best pieces of exercise equipment: the doorframe pull-up bar.

In order to understand why I'd write a book focused on a single piece of equipment, it's important to know a bit about my background in the fitness world. My journey began in 2002 when I decided to become a personal trainer. Initially, I did it simply to learn how to improve my own workouts while making a few extra dollars on the side. I quickly fell in love with fitness as I grew passionate about understanding how the body works and the different ways that one could effect change on it. Like most trainers, I started my career working at a couple of large health clubs. That experience allowed me to train a diverse clientele base, as well as work with and learn from some brilliant minds in the fitness industry. I eventually moved on to start my own business, My Home Trainer, a personal training company that sends trainers to the client's home. Working in this setting forced me to make the most of my surroundings and allowed me to test my own creativity.

Variety is important in developing an exercise program because it keeps things interesting and allows a person to make progress. Working in a health club gives a trainer access to hundreds of unique pieces of equipment. When working at home, there's typically very limited access to equipment, and I quickly learned that a person had to make the most out of a small number of items in order to both achieve results and stave off boredom. This is where I discovered the value of the doorframe pull-up bar. For me it killed two birds with one stone: It supplied enough diversity to keep the workouts progressive and different, and also provided enough of a challenge to impart consistent and great results.

Of the many benefits of the doorframe pull-up bar, the one that stands out the most is the ability to perform pull-ups almost anywhere. Pull-ups are in the opinion of many, myself included, the very best exercise. Having this as an option while training my clients in a limited setting allows them to achieve significant results. I've had great success with my in-home clients, largely due to the diversity of the doorframe pull-up bar and the ability to perform pull-ups combined with other key exercises.

For years, pull-ups have been a staple in my own workouts as well as my clients' and I've seen great results in both areas. *Doorframe Pull-Up Bar Workouts* is my chance to share simple, no-frills, goal-oriented workouts that are useful for any number of goals, including weight loss, functional strength, athletic conditioning, core stability and increased muscle tone.

If you're one of the many who find pull-ups intimidating, too difficult or impossible to attain, don't worry. Included is a program designed to help you build up to performing pull-ups. Additionally, there are many modifications described in this book that will assist you in getting many of the benefits of pull-ups, even if you can't yet perform a full one.

While I'm a big proponent of pull-ups, what makes the doorframe pull-up bar even more effective is that you can perform other exercises with it. You can use it for hanging ab movements to work the midsection and core. Additionally, it can be placed on the floor for upper- and lower-body exercises. I find using a doorframe pull-up bar in combination with bodyweight exercises to be among the most effective and efficient ways to exercise.

My goal is that you find this book to be accessible and valuable regardless of your fitness level. Total beginners will have access to step-by-step instructions on the core movements as well as valuable information that anyone starting an exercise program should have. If you suffer from a muscular or joint injury or limitation, I provide detailed instructions on how to modify movements in order to get the benefits of exercise without exacerbating an injury. If you're more advanced or athletic, there are advanced workouts and exercises to maximize your results. If you're a fitness enthusiast looking to change things up, you'll find programs to help re-energize your fitness routine. No matter what your level, you'll find *Doorframe Pull-Up Bar Workouts* to be an essential part of your fitness library.

ABOUT THIS BOOK

Doorframe Pull-Up Bar Workouts has been designed to provide you with all of the information that you need to begin or expand on an exercise program in the comfort of your home. All you need is a doorframe pull-up bar and this book to achieve any number of goals and objectives.

This book consists of three sections. Part I talks about the doorframe pull-up bar in detail and explains the fundamentals of exercise and fitness. Part II takes you through fitness testing and baseline assessments, useful if you'd like to measure your progress. It also contains a variety of preset programs and describes how to design your own. The programs are all based on goals, so you'll have the opportunity to select a program that specifically caters to your needs.

Part III is made up of all the exercises, with options for making them harder or easier. If you're comfortable designing your own exercise programs, you can skip right to this section. The appendix provides you with movements for warming up and cooling down, as well as stretches.

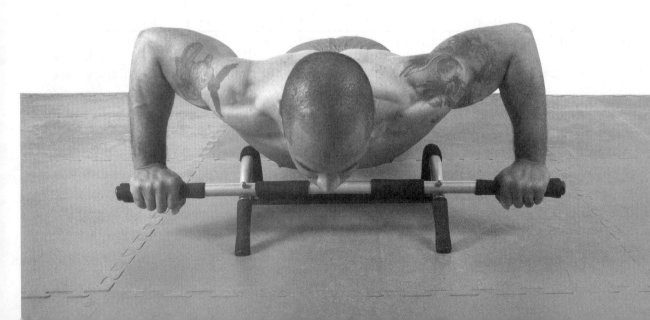

THE DOORFRAME PULL-UP BAR

WHAT IS THE DOORFRAME PULL-UP BAR?

If you purchase one piece of exercise equipment for your home, it should be the doorframe pull-up bar. The most practical and efficient solution to installing a pull-up bar in the home, it's easy to find and can be purchased online or at any sporting goods store.

There are many options when deciding on a doorframe pull-up system. Companies like Iron Gym and Waccess offer systems that require no major installation, although they do need molding on a doorframe. Basically, they hook around one side of a doorframe and use the handles on the other side to evenly distribute the weight. They're safe and sturdy and can be set up and taken down in a matter of seconds. Their small size also makes them portable and easy to carry around.

Doorframe pull-up bars have the added bonus of working as a floor unit and can be used for a wide variety of floor exercises, which I discuss later in this book. Iron Gym and Astone Fitness also offer "extreme" versions, which offer many more positions to grip the bar. Their angled ends provide a slightly better hand position for performing wide-grip pull-ups.

WHY THE DOORFRAME PULL-UP BAR?

Throughout my career as a fitness professional, I've had the opportunity to work in a variety of settings. I've worked out of huge luxury fitness centers, small recreation centers and tiny NYC apartments. I've worked in settings with the newest and most advanced equipment, and I've trained clients in the park. Over time I discovered that, somewhat counterintuitively, I saw better results with the clients who had minimal equipment. The lack of equipment in these settings meant that my workouts were based almost exclusively on bodyweight exercises. As these clients increased their strength and adapted to the various exercises, I was forced to push the envelope and make things more challenging and dynamic. In many cases, their functional strength and ability went through the roof because we didn't have the equipment at a traditional gym to fall back on. More often than not, pull-ups were at the center of these exercise programs, and this is what really sold me on the value of the doorframe pull-up bar.

The doorframe pull-up bar is incredibly diverse and has quite a few significant benefits.

1 EASE OF USE: In the not-so-distant past, setting up a home pull-up bar meant permanently installing a bar in your home. While this may work if you have a dedicated exercise space, it presents a challenge if you don't want a pull-up bar hanging at all times. There's also the issue of actually installing a bar that can support hundreds of pounds of weight. The doorframe pull-up bar solves these problems because it literally takes seconds to set up and requires no installation.

2 PORTABILITY: The doorframe pull-up bar can be taken apart in less than a minute and stored away easily. You can then pack it up and take it with you to work or when traveling.

3 VARIETY OF EXERCISES: The doorframe pull-up bar allows for a wide range of exercises, including dozens of pull-ups and variations, hanging abdominal exercises and floor exercises that can all be performed with only the doorframe pull-up bar.

4 CENTER OF A HOME-BASED EXERCISE PROGRAM: Because the doorframe pull-up bar allows for pull-ups, it's perfect for a home-based fitness program and can be as effective as working out in a fully equipped facility.

BENEFITS OF EXERCISING AT HOME	BENEFITS OF THE DOORFRAME PULL-UP BAR	BENEFITS OF PULL-UPS
▪ Saves time	▪ Portable	▪ Multi-joint exercise
▪ Saves money	▪ Easy set-up and take-down	▪ Build strength
▪ Nonjudgmental environment	▪ No installation	▪ Functional
▪ Play your own music	▪ Multiple grips	▪ Improve athletic ability
▪ Bodyweight exercises are mostly compound movements	▪ Floor exercises	
▪ Train on your own schedule		

WHY PULL-UPS?

The very mention of pull-ups tends to generate a reaction unlike any other exercise. For some it's a sense of dread. For others, it brings back bad memories of elementary school gym class. There are those who see them as a source of strength and empowerment, and then there are those who view pull-ups as a goal or a milestone that they'd one day like to attain. In my career as a personal trainer, pull-ups have been by far the most common exercise mentioned as a goal.

Pull-ups have these kinds of reactions, and many more, because they're very hard. Actively pulling your entire bodyweight off of the ground is a great demonstration of strength and indicator of athletic ability, so much that they're a staple of physical fitness testing for professional athletics and the military.

Personally, pull-ups have played an extremely important role in my own strength-training program. I was a big weightlifter well into my 20s. In my late 20s, I decided to begin and eventually compete in Muay Thai, a martial art originating in Thailand. I fell in love with the sport but found that when I combined it with traditional weight training, I was constantly getting injured, so I needed to find a way to maintain my strength without getting hurt. That's when I turned to pull-ups and other bodyweight exercises. It worked wonders, as I was able to maintain and even increase my strength while staying healthy. Pull-ups have been an integral part of my own training regimen ever since.

There are plenty of reasons why pull-ups are a great exercise. First, they're easy to set up. With the doorframe pull-up bar, it's possible to put up a pull-up bar almost anywhere with little to no installation. It's especially good for tiny apartments. Additionally, the movement itself is fairly simple (although note that I didn't say easy): You grab a bar and pull yourself up until your chin is over the bar.

Pull-ups are a great strength-building compound exercise; multiple joints and muscles work together to produce the movement. Additionally, pull-ups require you to stabilize your entire body, which means much greater neuromuscular recruitment. This builds functional strength as you're forced to completely control what your body does with no external assistance. Pull-ups are also great for grip strength, and that alone has applications in a wide variety of sports and activities.

Another great thing about pull-ups is how variable they truly are. While a traditional pull-up is difficult, the movement can be modified to meet the needs of someone struggling with it. Alternatively, there are many ways to make the traditional pull-up progressively harder in order to maintain its difficulty. Thus, some kind of pull-up can be performed by almost anyone participating in a fitness program.

WHAT IF I CAN'T DO PULL-UPS?

Don't worry. There's a program specifically designed to build up to full pull-ups. I've also included plenty of modifications so you'll still get many of the benefits while you work toward developing your pull-ups.

THE MUSCLES

The combination of a doorframe pull-up bar and bodyweight exercises can target all of the major muscles and muscle groups throughout the body. This means that you can get a complete and total-body workout anywhere. The doorframe pull-up bar is especially effective in working the lats, upper back and biceps, which can be difficult to target with a traditional bodyweight training routine.

While this isn't a complete list of the muscles and their functions, I've tried to briefly cover muscles that are commonly focused on with exercise.

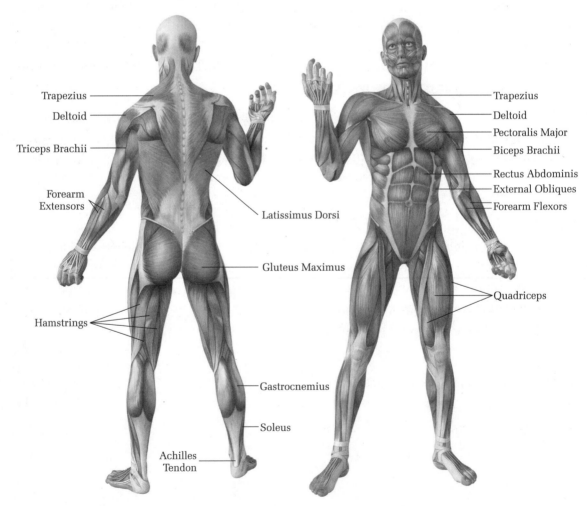

Trapezius

Deltoid

Triceps Brachii

Forearm Extensors

Latissimus Dorsi

Gluteus Maximus

Hamstrings

Gastrocnemius

Soleus

Achilles Tendon

Trapezius

Deltoid

Pectoralis Major

Biceps Brachii

Rectus Abdominis

External Obliques

Forearm Flexors

Quadriceps

LATISSIMUS DORSI (LATS): The broadest muscle in the back, responsible for extension and abduction of the shoulder joint. It's the primary muscle used when performing pull-ups.

PECTORALIS MAJOR (CHEST): A large muscle situated on the chest, it's responsible for flexion and horizontal adduction at the shoulder joint. It's the primary muscle when performing push-ups.

DELTOIDS (SHOULDER): The muscle formed around the shoulder consists of three distinct heads: anterior deltoid, lateral deltoid and posterior deltoid. The deltoids are responsible for abduction, flexion and extension of the shoulder joint.

BICEPS BRACHII (BICEPS): The muscle on the anterior (front) of the arm, it's responsible for flexion at the elbow joint.

TRICEPS BRACHII (TRICEPS): The muscle on the posterior (rear) part of the arm, it's responsible for extension at the elbow joint.

TRAPEZIUS (TRAPS): The large muscle located on the upper back, it's responsible for retraction of the scapulae (shoulder blades) and elevation of the shoulder.

RHOMBOID MAJOR (RHOMBOIDS): An important muscle located in the upper back, it's responsible for retracting the scapulae (shoulder blades).

RECTUS ABDOMINIS (ABS OR ABDOMINALS): The "six-pack" muscle, this long muscle located on the trunk is responsible for flexion and assists in stabilization of the trunk.

INTERNAL/EXTERNAL OBLIQUES (OBLIQUES): The muscles located on the sides of the trunk, these are responsible for rotation and lateral flexion of the trunk. They also assist in trunk flexion and stabilization.

ERECTOR SPINAE (LOWER BACK): Muscles located on the back, they're responsible for extension of the trunk.

PSOAS MAJOR (HIP FLEXORS): Located between the lower spine and the top of the thigh, this muscle is responsible for flexion and lateral rotation at the hip.

GLUTEALS (GLUTES): Consisting of the gluteus maximus, gluteus medius and gluteus minimus, these muscles are responsible for extension, abduction and lateral rotation at the hip.

QUADRICEPS (QUADS): Located on the front of the thigh, these muscles are responsible for knee extension.

HAMSTRINGS: Located on the back of the thigh, these muscles are responsible for knee flexion, hip extension and external rotation at the hip.

ADDUCTORS (GROIN): These muscles located on the inner thigh are responsible for adduction of the legs.

CALVES: Consisting of the gastrocnemius and the soleus, the calves are the muscle in the back of the lower leg. They're responsible for plantar flexion of the foot (pointing the toes away from the knee).

TIBIALIS ANTERIOR (SHIN): This muscle along the front of the lower leg is responsible for dorsiflexion (pointing the toes toward the knee).

CORE: The core is a combination of muscles that work together to stabilize the trunk. These muscles include the rectus abdominis, obliques, erector spinae and psoas, among many others.

UPPER BACK: This refers to muscles that assist in stabilizing and retracting the shoulder blades. Muscles include the trapezius, rhomboids and posterior deltoid, among others.

FOREARMS: This refers to the muscles of the lower part of the arm. It includes the wrist flexors, wrist extensors and supinator. The forearms play a large role in stabilizing the body during pull-ups.

COMPONENTS OF A MOVEMENT

The components of a movement are important but commonly overlooked parts of exercise. Understanding these components as well as the variables associated with them is the key to designing an effective fitness program. These are important things to be aware of as they apply to every exercise.

All exercise involves some combination of concentric, eccentric and isometric action. When participating in a strength-training program, we should be aware of the different components and how they'll affect movements.

CONCENTRIC MUSCLE CONTRACTION (POSITIVE): A concentric muscle contraction is one in which the muscle increases tension and shortens. This type of action occurs when we exert force against an object and we overcome the object's weight or resistance. Concentric contractions are easy to identify in bodyweight training—any movement that moves the body up against gravity is a result of concentric action.

ECCENTRIC MUSCLE CONTRACTION (NEGATIVE): An eccentric muscle contraction is one in which the muscle increases tension as it lengthens. Unlike a concentric contraction, the force that we exert over the object, or resistance, is not enough to overcome it, leading to muscle lengthening. Eccentric contractions are easy to identify in bodyweight training—any movement in which your body moves down with gravity is a result of eccentric action.

ISOMETRIC MUSCLE CONTRACTION (STATIC): An isometric muscle contraction is one in which muscle tension increases but the muscle remains static—there's no lengthening or shortening of the muscle. In these cases, the force being exerted is equal to the object's weight or resistance.

Using the standard pull-up as an example, concentric action occurs when we pull ourselves up. We're exerting force (our bodyweight) against an object and overcoming it. Isometric action occurs at the top of the movement when we pause. At this stage, we're exerting just enough force to stay at that position. Eccentric action occurs as we lower ourselves down to end the pull-up. In this case, we exert enough force to maintain control over the movement but our weight overcomes the force.

BRACING THE CORE: The muscles that make up the core act like a belt to stabilize the spine during exercise. The core should be engaged during most exercises, especially those in which you're susceptible to arching your back. The technique for engaging your core is called "abdominal bracing." The goal is to tighten all of the trunk muscles, thereby stabilizing the spine. You do this by bracing the trunk as if you were bracing for a punch. When you do this, you should feel your trunk tighten around you.

BREATHING: Breathing is often overlooked with exercise, and incorrect breathing can impair an exercise routine. When performing traditional strength or resistance exercises, exhale on the concentric portion; this helps to contract the diaphragm, adding additional stability to the trunk. When working with bodyweight, exhale when moving up. You should inhale on the eccentric portion. When working with bodyweight, this would be any movement going down. If you're performing an isometric movement, very fast repetitions or cardio, focus on controlled and consistent breathing. Instead of trying to time your breath with movements, try to inhale for 1–2 seconds and exhale for 1–2 seconds.

VARIABLES

Once you've decided on a movement, a group of variables will help determine a large part of the movement's training effect. Understanding how these variables apply to movements will help you understand the programs listed in this book as well as help you to design your own workouts or modify existing ones.

RANGE OF MOTION (ROM): The normal distance that a joint can move. Generally it's advisable to exercise through a normal range of motion; however, there some exceptions. A shortened ROM may be recommended as a way to make an exercise easier, when training for speed or if there's some kind of injury or limitation within the joint.

REPETITIONS (REPS): One repetition is any movement in which you begin in one position, produce a movement and return back to the initial position. Using a squat as an example, if the starting position is standing up, one repetition would be completed once you sit back and extend up to the standing position again.

SETS: A set is a series of consecutive repetitions. As an example, 1 set of 10 repetitions of squats would be completed once you perform 10 consecutive squats.

TEMPO: The speed of the movement. Tempo usually consists of three numbers, referring to the number of seconds to perform the concentric, isometric and eccentric actions. As an example, if you're performing a pull-up, a tempo of 1-1-3 would mean that the pulling-up portion should be done in 1 second, the isometric hold at the top of the movement should be held for 1 second, and the lowering portion should be completed over 3 seconds.

The tempo should be even and consistent throughout the exercise's ROM. If, for example, the eccentric portion is 5 seconds, that should be spread along the entire range and not predominantly during the top or bottom portion. A slower tempo, especially on the eccentric portion, will result in greater muscular tension and lead to greater strength and muscular gains. A faster tempo functions better for speed, endurance and conditioning training. Some exercises, speed squats for example, require you to use momentum throughout the movement. These exercises will typically be performed at a shorter ROM and your aim should be to complete them as quickly as you can. A ballistic movement, like a full-body push-up, differs from momentum in that the focus is to complete the concentric portion of the exercise as powerfully as possible.

INTENSITY: A measurement of how much energy is expended during an exercise or a workout. There are two ways to measure intensity. The first is by your heart rate. The second is by determining your rate of perceived exertion (RPE). To measure your RPE, gauge how you feel on a scale of 1–10, with 1 being completely at rest and 10 being a level of intensity that you would not be able to keep up for more than a few seconds. Measuring your RPE is more common during aerobic activity and conditioning programs. When strength training, the general rule is that the last one to two repetitions should be difficult. Your intensity will determine the amount of time you need to exercise. A high-intensity program requires less time and is more efficient.

RPE SCALE		
RATING	*PERCEPTION*	*ACTIVITY*
0–1	Very light	Watching TV
2–3	Light	Light housework
4–5	Moderate	Dancing
6–7	Hard/ Vigorous	Jogging
8–9	Very Hard	Running
10	Maximal	All-out sprint

LOAD: Any external resistance. Since this book focuses on the doorframe pull-up bar, your bodyweight is the only external resistance. If you wanted to increase the load, a weight vest or weighted backpack would suffice.

REST: The amount of time you take to rest between exercises. Rest can vary from a couple of seconds up to 5 minutes for very heavy strength training. Heavy resistance training will typically require longer rest than other forms of exercise. Shorter rest periods allow you to train your recovery time and to get more work done over shorter periods of time. You can manipulate these variables as you see fit in order to get the most out of your workout. Whether you're designing your own program, following one of the many in this book or modifying an existing program, these are the key components to any exercise.

WHAT IS FITNESS?

When we think about fitness, we usually associate it with being in good physical health and of sound body and mind. My favorite definition, however, is simply one's ability to efficiently complete a given task. It's a broad definition, but one that captures the subjectivity as well as the complexity of fitness.

Fitness is relative. It's based on the individual, and the necessary components are specific to the task at hand. A marathon runner and an amateur wrestler would both be considered fit, but the specific components are going to be completely different for each athlete. A marathon runner needs to be able to produce constant lower-intensity energy over a very long period of time. An amateur wrestler needs to produce high-intensity movements in short bursts over a much shorter period of time. As you can see, these are two different tasks that require different components of fitness. We also have to look at the individual in order to determine what qualifies as good fitness. An elite athlete is going to have different requirements for fitness than a person recovering from hip replacement surgery. These individual differences mean that each person has to look at their own lifestyle, abilities and goals in order to determine what fitness means to them.

In a reductive sense, fitness is about disease prevention and the ability to perform normal daily activities. In order to measure one's fitness, we look at three different components. First is *cardiovascular ability*. This essentially refers to your ability to efficiently extract oxygen from the blood. Second is *functional ability*. This is your body's ability to perform normal movements without pain or restrictions. Third is *muscular strength*. This refers to the amount of force that you can apply in a given movement. In addition to the three that I've mentioned, mental health and diet are also very important. Each one can have a significant impact on one's fitness level, both positive and negative. Each of these categories can then be broken down even further, but this is what we look at in order to determine fitness.

EXERCISE

In order to maintain and improve our fitness levels, we need to exercise. Like fitness, the definition of exercise is broad, encompassing anything that requires an energy expenditure greater than normal daily activities. One great thing is that exercise covers a wide variety of activities. You don't have to be in a gym working with dumbbells, machines and treadmills to be exercising. Exercise can be dynamic, as long as you're working hard.

The human body is an amazingly adaptive machine. If you apply stress to your body, it will do everything that it can to handle the stress and it will respond by adapting to deal with it more efficiently in the future. This is essentially how we improve our fitness level — we stress the body with some form of exercise. The body then responds by adapting to the stress by repairing itself stronger than it was in order to handle the new level of stress. Benefits of exercises are:

- Increases strength

- Increases endurance

- Decreases body fat

- Helps fight disease

- Lowers blood pressure

- Increases mood

- Increases cognitive ability

- Improves self-esteem

- Increases energy levels

While the definition of fitness may be broad, there are some basic recommendations that everyone should follow to be healthy. According to the American College of Sports Medicine, these are the weekly minimum recommendations for exercise:

WEEKLY MINIMUM FITNESS RECOMMENDATIONS	
AEROBIC ACTIVITY	150 minutes of moderate-intensity activity OR 80 minutes of vigorous activity
STRENGTH TRAINING	Train every muscle group 2–3 days
FLEXIBILITY TRAINING	2–3 days
FUNCTIONAL TRAINING	2–3 days

While these represent the minimum recommendations, it's actually very flexible. Much of the functional training can be incorporated into the resistance training, especially when you incorporate bodyweight exercises into your fitness routine. Additionally, the aerobic activity can be completed in either multiple short bursts or in fewer longer sessions. Even if you can't meet the minimum recommendations, you can still benefit greatly from exercise.

Beyond the general recommendations, there's what's considered to be performance-based fitness. Performance-based fitness extends beyond general fitness because these goals are more specific, varying widely from sports-related training to weight loss to physique training to post-rehab. In these cases, the fitness components become more specific, which means that the exercise programs have to be more detailed.

COMPONENTS OF A HEALTHY LIFESTYLE

Healthy living requires a combination of lifestyle choices. While exercise is incredibly important, it's crucial to manage other aspects of your life in order to achieve optimal health, fitness and performance. Each component has an effect on all of the others, so if any one component is subpar, it will bring down all of the others.

1 RESISTANCE TRAINING: This form of exercise uses an external resistance (including one's bodyweight) in order to build strength. Benefits include muscular size and strength, and increased bone density.

2 CARDIOVASCULAR TRAINING: This lower-intensity, longer-duration exercise uses oxygen for energy. Benefits include fighting disease, lowering blood pressure, decreasing body composition and weight loss.

3 FUNCTIONAL TRAINING: This movement-based training focuses on developing, enhancing and strengthening specific movement patterns. Benefits include better balance, more fluid movements and increased sport-specific skills.

4 FLEXIBILITY: These exercises are based on developing the optimal range of motion within a joint. Benefits include better posture and balance between muscles, and reduced chance of injuries.

5 DIET: A good diet helps in a variety of ways. Diet is important if you have a specific weight-loss or weight-gain goal. Additionally, healthy eating will help significantly to reduce the risk of a variety of diseases. Eating the right foods can both enhance performance during exercise and aid in recovery.

6 WATER: Drinking the right amount of water will maintain hydration levels and enhance performance. Additionally, it helps with energy levels and regulates body temperature.

7 SLEEP: Getting a good amount of sleep will help to reduce stress, increase energy and aid in recovery.

MISCONCEPTIONS

Exercise, health and fitness is still a developing and constantly changing field of research. Almost weekly, new trends, studies, products and programs emerge that seem to contradict previous knowledge. With so much information available, it can be difficult to separate facts from fallacies. The following are some common fitness misconceptions that have been proven to be false.

THE MISCONCEPTION: Women have to train differently from men.

THE REALITY: The physiological response to exercise is the same between men and women, although men have a higher testosterone level and lower gender-specific fat, which allows them to respond to exercise faster in many cases. When developing an exercise program, the focus should be on goals, not on gender.

THE MISCONCEPTION: Low-intensity cardio is better for fat loss.

THE REALITY: This is technically true in that low-intensity and long-duration cardio will use a higher percentage of fat for energy, but it's highly inefficient. A higher-intensity cardio program has many more health and fitness benefits. First, you'll burn more total calories in a significantly shorter amount of time. Second, a higher-intensity program will boost your metabolism, meaning that your body will continue to burn calories even at rest. A higher-intensity cardio program is far more effective for weight loss and conditioning.

THE MISCONCEPTION: Post-exercise soreness is a sign of a good workout. If I'm not sore, I didn't work hard enough.

THE REALITY: This is a very common misconception about a common thing that happens for a variety of reasons. It's most common when starting an exercise program or when trying something new. One important thing to note: Soreness is not an indicator of a tough workout. You should judge your workout based on how much effort you put into it. If you feel like your workout is challenging in the moment, then that should be enough.

THE MISCONCEPTION: I'm not working hard enough if I'm not sweating.

THE REALITY: The purpose of perspiration, or sweat, is to cool the body down. When we exercise, our body temperature rises, so sweating normally occurs during exercise. Every individual is different and some people sweat a lot with minimal activity, while others can go through an incredibly intense workout with minimal perspiration. You should judge the difficulty of your workout based on how you feel, not by how much you're sweating.

THE MISCONCEPTION: If I wear a sweat suit while I exercise, I'll burn more fat.

THE REALITY: This can be very dangerous. Sweat suits are useful for athletes that need to make weight for competition (like wrestlers and boxers) but are of little use to everyone else. You sweat in order to cool the body down and keep it from overheating. Wearing a sweat suit causes the body to overheat and in turn sweat more. As a result, you risk heat stroke, dehydration and kidney damage. Additionally, there's no additional fat loss while wearing a sweat suit, and any weight loss will come back as soon as you rehydrate.

THE MISCONCEPTION: There are separate upper and lower abs.

THE REALITY: This is one of the most persistent myths out there. The rectus abdominis (the six-pack muscle) is one long muscle connecting at the rib cage and at the pelvis. A combination of connective and fibrous tissue gives it the six-pack look. The rectus abdominis acts as one muscle in that it either contracts as a whole or it doesn't. There are some exercises which will place slightly more emphasis on one portion over the other, but it's not possible to isolate the upper and lower halves.

THE MISCONCEPTION: The more time I spend exercising, the better my results will be.

THE REALITY: Efficiency is the key to fitness. It's generally better to work at a high intensity for a shorter period of time than it is to work at a low intensity for a longer period. You can get an awesome workout in 10 minutes if you work hard enough.

THE MISCONCEPTION: I need to do lots of crunches in order to have a flat and defined stomach (spot reduction).

THE REALITY: Muscle definition in any area is a combination of low body fat and muscle. Exercises, like crunches, will help to develop the muscle but will do little to burn fat. To lose the fat, you'll need a combination of aerobic activity and a clean diet. Additionally, regarding fat loss, you can't pick and chose where and how your body loses it.

THE MISCONCEPTION: In order to tone up, I need to lift lighter weights for high reps.

THE REALITY: The idea of "toning up" is a bit of a misconception in itself. Muscle tone technically refers to the normal unconscious activation of muscles. Our muscles are always minimally activated in order to maintain posture and to be able to react quickly if needed. What people mean when they refer to "tone" is actually muscle definition. Even if we substitute the words, the phrase is still a misconception. Definition, sculpting, toning or whatever you want to call it is achieved by a combination of low body fat and increased muscle mass. High-repetition exercise is good for muscle endurance but not for definition. In order to develop definition, you need to engage in a combination of fat-burning activities (cardiovascular training, healthy eating) and muscle-building activities (strength training).

THE MISCONCEPTION: I sit in an office all day, but since I exercise five days a week for an hour, I'm not sedentary.

THE REALITY: Recent research strongly suggests that even if you exceed the minimum activity requirements, you can still suffer from the effects of a sedentary lifestyle. As it turns out, engaging in exercise and being sedentary are mutually exclusive. If you spend too much time seated without getting up and moving around, you can suffer all of the negative effects of being sedentary. Ideally, you should get up and move around every 20–30 minutes.

THE MISCONCEPTION: It's best to exercise in the morning.

THE REALITY: The "best" time to exercise is whatever time works best for you. One of the most important aspects of a fitness program is making it fit into your life while creating minimal stress. This means that you should schedule your workouts at a time that's convenient and that you can commit to. The one caveat here is that, from experience, people who exercise in the morning tend to be the most consistent. This is because it takes discipline to exercise first thing in the morning. Second, if you can exercise early, you're unlikely to face many of the distractions and obstacles that pop up as the day moves on.

THE MISCONCEPTION: I'm overweight — I need to focus on cardio before strength training.

THE REALITY: Even if your primary goal is weight loss, you can still derive great results from strength training. Strength training will help you build muscle. That muscle will help to increase your metabolism, which means that you'll be burning more calories at rest. Increasing your resting metabolic rate will help significantly with weight loss over time.

THE MISCONCEPTION: I should stretch before I exercise.

THE REALITY: In most cases, stretching is best left for the end of your workout. While stretching has an overall positive effect on fitness, stretching immediately before exercise has been shown to increase the risk of injury. Stretching before exercise is recommended in some situations, such as if you have a muscle or joint tightness; doing so may be necessary to increase your range of motion. Additionally, if you participate in a sport or activity that may push the limits of your flexibility, pre-exercise stretching may be recommended.

THE MISCONCEPTION: Lactic acid build-up is what causes pain during and after intense exercise.

THE REALITY: This is the misconception that won't go away. Lactic acid, or lactate, is actually a good thing. In response to intense exercise, the body reacts by producing lactate from glucose as a source of fuel for the muscles. Additionally, the pain after exercise is actually due to small microscopic tears in the muscle.

KEYS TO SUCCESS

Your approach to fitness is just as important as the actual components of your fitness program. The success of a workout program is often determined by your level of preparation in addition to how well you integrate fitness into your lifestyle. Exercise is a necessity and it should be looked at as a part of your life. Much like eating, showering and brushing teeth, at a minimum exercise should be a part of life that occurs in regular intervals. Obviously exercise requires more time, preparation and physical exertion than the other examples, but it's no less important or necessary.

Most people aren't passionate about the process of actually exercising. We're all aware of the benefits and we love the results but, for most people, the process leaves much to be desired. Devoting three to six hours a week to any activity can be difficult, so the challenge is to find a way of integrating fitness into your life as seamlessly as possible. The process of integration involves four steps that will help you lay the foundation for a solid fitness program.

STEP 1: GOAL SETTING

Goal setting is an important component to sustaining a fitness program. By doing so, we give ourselves something to work toward and aspire to. This increases motivation since there's a clear objective. This is especially true if you're not in love with the exercise itself. It's common for a person to begin a fitness program and see results initially but over time become bored or frustrated with any lack of progress. Oftentimes, this happens because, while the person is still making progress, they're not actively measuring it. It's important that the goals be measurable because sometimes we can't see or feel the progress until we can objectively identify it.

Assessment and reassessment (fitness testing and retesting) are key components to goal setting. An initial assessment will give you a baseline to work with and reassessments will allow you to measure your progress and modify your goals. The timing of your reassessments is also important. You should allow for enough time to pass that you'll see reasonable progress, but not so much time that you lose sight of the goals. Typically, assessing/reassessing every four to eight weeks is reasonable. Tracking progress like this keeps you aware of and motivated to achieve your goals.

It's important to have immediate, short- and long-term goals. *Immediate goals* are typically within one to two weeks and usually represent workout-related goals. An immediate goal may be to exercise five times in the week or to perform 12 pull-ups during a particular workout session. *Short-term goals* are typically within one to three months. These goals are usually related to your assessment and reassessment. Examples would be losing inches on your waist, building your biceps or improving your body composition. *Long-term goals* are typically between six months to one year and beyond; they represent the ultimate goal or objective of your fitness program.

Mixing these three kinds of goals can really help to keep you on track. Having a long-term goal is very important, but often the time frame is too long to keep a person motivated. By having medium- and short-term goals, too, you can see progress in smaller blocks and you'll feel a sense of accomplishment as you chip away at the ultimate goal.

Another important reason for goal setting and assessment is that you're able to identify problems and make appropriate adjustments to your exercise program. If you reassess every six weeks, you can modify your program if you're not seeing the progress that you'd like. If you don't check regularly, you can plateau for months without knowing for sure. Six months to a year down the road, it can be incredibly frustrating and discouraging to feel like you've made no progress.

STEP 2: REALISTIC OUTLOOK

It's always important to ask yourself, "What are my goals and why?" The "why" is essential because you should have a realistic outlook when it comes to both your exercise program and your goals. It's important to understand the risks of trying for too much too quickly.

One of your ultimate goals should be to incorporate exercise and fitness into your lifestyle. For most people, this means balancing exercise with work, friends, hobbies and family obligations. In this case, finding a routine that's minimally invasive is far more important than finding the perfect routine.

It's important to understand that the more extreme the goal, the greater the potential to fall off. An extreme goal means a complete lifestyle change and a commitment to diet and exercise that's far beyond what's normal. In most cases, the huge change proves to be too much and there's a complete drop-off. I've seen people begin a program, lose 20 pounds in two months and then quickly gain everything back because the change was simply too much of a shock.

Sometimes you'll have a specific goal that requires a significant change. A wedding or a marathon can represent something that would require a serious commitment. While this can provide great motivation, it's important to know how difficult the training will be and to have a maintenance plan in place once you've reached that goal. If you get into great shape for your wedding, it would be a shame to not have a plan in place to maintain the progress that you've made.

STEP 3: ACCOUNTABILITY

Finding ways to hold yourself accountable will help to keep fitness in the forefront. The purpose of holding yourself accountable isn't to make you feel guilty or to punish you, but rather to make sure you're always actively aware of your current fitness program.

The key to holding yourself accountable is that you're aware of and acknowledge your fitness routine regardless of whether it's going well or you're slacking off. I've found a variety of strategies to be successful, so use the methods that work best for you.

KEEP A JOURNAL: A fitness journal can be as detailed or as simple as you'd like. You can track every bit of data or just write two sentences. The key here is that you write every day. This way, even when you miss a workout, you have to acknowledge it.

WORK OUT WITH A FRIEND: Having a workout partner is great because you can be accountable to each other. Sometimes having another person can be more fun and motivating.

USE A FITNESS TRACKING DEVICE: There are currently a lot of great devices on the market that you can use to track your activity. Devices like UP by Jawbone and Fitbit are great options. They allow you to track your activity levels on a daily basis in a way that's non-invasive but requires your attention.

COMPETE WITH YOURSELF: When you exercise, make it a competition between your present self and your past self. Whenever you exercise, your objective should be to perform a little bit better than you performed during your last workout.

REWARD YOURSELF FOR REACHING MILESTONES: Among the goals that you set for yourself, there'll be certain milestones that represent significant progress. The goals should represent a more long-term goal like exercising consistently for six months, improving from 3 to 20 consecutive pull-ups or losing 30 pounds. When you reach these milestones, reward yourself with something.

STEP 4: ELIMINATE OBSTACLES AND EXCUSES

Life has a way of throwing more than enough obstacles in the way of even the most passionate of fitness enthusiasts. The ability to anticipate and plan around potential obstacles is a significant aspect of maintaining a consistent fitness program. List any obstacles that you may encounter in your day-to-day life and find ways to work your fitness routine around them. Below, I've listed common obstacles and some potential strategies to avoid them.

TIME: Time is the single biggest obstacle when it comes to maintaining a consistent exercise program. Work, family and social obligations can easily take over a person's life and it's often at the expense of their fitness. Time doesn't need to be a problem at all. Having the option to exercise at home saves the precious time that you'd need to get to and from the gym. Additionally, when using a program like high-intensity interval training (HIIT), you can get a complete workout in10–20 minutes or less, saving significant time.

MONEY: Money is another common obstacle, and it's often tied to the misconception that you need a gym to get into shape. The great thing about fitness is that you need little more than your body and some creativity. This book provides everything you need to get a great workout without ever setting foot in a gym.

STRESS: Stress can come in many forms and often leads to a serious aversion to exercise. Ironically, exercise can serve as a great form of stress relief. If you feel like you're too stressed to exercise, then try to start slowly. Begin with a lighter workout simply to establish some consistency. Over time, you should find that while stress may keep you from beginning the workout, once you start, the exercise will actually make you feel better.

INJURY/ILLNESS: Injuries and illnesses can be difficult to deal with for a variety of reasons. The first step is to speak with your doctor or physical therapist to advise you on what movements and types of exercise you can and can't do. Regardless of the injury or illness, exercise is still necessary for almost everyone, so it's important to develop ways to work around them.

Excuses are different from obstacles in that they're usually used as a way to rationalize not exercising. Common excuses include:

BOREDOM: If you use the same routine day to day and week to week, it's easy for boredom to set in. To combat this, change things up by trying new exercises and progressing on current ones. You can also try new programs. This book has a lot of options, so you should never have to deal with boredom.

FRUSTRATION DUE TO A LACK OF PROGRESS: If you feel like you're not making progress, make sure that you're properly assessing and reassessing. Sometimes we focus on one variable without seeing the whole picture. Weight is a common variable that gets over-emphasized. It's not uncommon for a person's weight to remain the same while they lose body fat, gain muscle and lose inches around the waist. If you're frustrated, change things up. There's enough variety in this book to keep you going for a long time.

NEGATIVE ATTITUDE TOWARD FITNESS: Many people simply dislike exercise and use that as an excuse to skip working out. If you fall into this category, it's important to figure out the source. Is it because you dislike physical exertion? Did you have a bad past experience in a gym? Once you identify the source of the aversion you can take steps to correct the problem. Exercise is not as rigid as it can be made out to be. Find an activity that provides the least resistance and stress. Try to be consistent and maximize your time.

Fitness can be fun, rewarding and life changing. You should always try to maintain a positive attitude and outlook. You don't necessarily have to love exercise, but the right approach and a positive attitude will help you navigate the highs and lows that come with any long-term project. If you slip up, try not to dwell on it—simply jump right back into your program and keep moving forward.

NUTRITION AND EATING STRATEGIES

Diet plays an important role in life and fitness. It's your primary source of energy and can enhance or diminish your performance. While you'll find the information in this section useful, it's important for me to clarify that I'm not a registered dietician. I have experience with performance-based nutrition but it's not my area of expertise, so this section will focus on general nutrition strategies. For most people, following these basic rules will be more than enough to allow your diet to complement your fitness program. If you have more specific dietary needs, I'd recommend meeting with a registered dietician.

Most of us have a love/hate relationship with food. It can provide the greatest of life's pleasures while at the same time creating limitless amounts of stress and anxiety. The key to a good diet, like exercise, is having the right approach. If you approach your diet with the proper mindset and preparation, then you'll significantly increase your chances of success.

DIET

Diet is literally and figuratively a four-letter word. It's one with a stigma attached to it. Simply speaking, the word conjures up thoughts of deprivation. Diets in the traditional sense are short term by design. They place your body in a state of starvation and you have no choice but to lose weight. The problem is that these diets aren't sustainable and at some point you'll have to stop. Most of the time, when a person stops a diet, they resort back to their previous habits and put the weight back on, and then some.

When I mention diet, I'm simply referring to the way that you eat and not a specific program. The reality is that a successful diet is one that doesn't make you miserable — it helps you achieve your fitness goals and is sustainable for life. Maintaining a successful diet is not without its challenges but, by following these simple rules, you can significantly increase your chances of success.

CALORIES IN VS. CALORIES OUT: Your daily caloric requirement (DCR) refers to the number of calories your body burns in a normal day. Once you determine your DCR, you can determine how many calories you need per day. If you want to lose weight, take in fewer calories than your DCR; if you want to gain weight, take in more calories. There are 3,500 calories in 1 pound of fat, so if your goal is to lose weight, you'd need to be at a caloric deficit of 500 per day in order to lose 1 pound of fat per week.

There are a couple of ways to determine your DCR. Easiest is to use an online calculator. Websites like ExRx.net are able to estimate your requirement based on numbers that you input. You can also do the math yourself. To do this, you first need to determine your basal metabolic rate (BMR), which is how many calories you burn per day completely at rest.

BMR for men = (12.7 x height in in.) + (6.23 x weight in lbs.)–(6.8 x age in yrs.) + 66

BMR for women = (4.7 x height in in.) + (4.35 x weight in lbs.)–(4.7 x age in yrs.) + 655

Once you've determined your BMR, the next step is to add your activity level to determine your DCR. Use the chart below to determine your activity level; multiply the number by your BMR to find your DCR.

DETERMINING YOUR DAILY CALORIC REQUIREMENT (DCR)	
LITTLE OR NO EXERCISE	BMR x 1.2
LIGHT EXERCISE 1–3 DAYS/WEEK	BMR x 1.375
MODERATE EXERCISE 3–5 DAYS/WEEK	BMR x 1.55
STRENUOUS EXERCISE 6–7 DAYS/WEEK	BMR x 1.725
PHYSICALLY STRENUOUS JOB OR 2 WORKOUTS A DAY	BMR x 1.9

Once you know your DCR, determine your target calories by adding or subtracting calories. For weight loss, a deficit of 500 calories per day will lead to 1 pound a week. So if your DCR is 2,000, your target calories would have to be 1,500 in order lose 1 pound a week.

The USDA has the following guidelines for caloric ratios: proteins, 10–35%; fats, 20–30%; carbohydrates: 45–55%.

PREPARATION: Preparation is incredibly important when it comes to a successful diet. We're far more likely to make poor decisions when we're hungry and unprepared. In these situations, it's much easier to give into cravings as well as to go for the easy option, both of which are usually unhealthy. You should do your best to plan your eating a week ahead of time. Try to anticipate any potential obstacles and have alternatives available. Plan ahead and avoid making food-related decisions when you're hungry.

EAT BREAKFAST: Eating breakfast helps stave off hunger throughout the day. This helps to fight cravings and poor food choices. Additionally, it provides you with a source of energy and structure for your diet.

DAY-TO-DAY CONSISTENCY: Try to find an eating schedule that you can maintain day to day. This will help with forming a routine. The goal is to develop a diet that's sustainable;

consistency will help make it second nature. If you have a solid and consistent routine, you're far more likely to bounce back if you slip up.

DRINK WATER: Drinking water is incredibly important. As we all know, humans can't survive more than a few days without water. It can help to increase performance when exercising since the muscles' cells need water to function properly. Water also helps to fight hunger, assists with the digestive process and regulates body temperature, among many other things. The general recommendation is to drink six to eight glasses a day. When exercising, amounts vary, but generally you should have an additional 8 ounces every 15 minutes. For more accuracy, you can weigh yourself post-workout and drink an additional 16 ounces for every pound lost.

CLEAN EATING: Try to keep your diet as clean as you can. Eat plenty of fruits, vegetables, whole grains and lean meats. Avoid processed foods, limit alcohol, salt, saturated fats and especially sugar. A clean diet will work wonders for your energy levels and your weight.

EAT 4 TO 6 TIMES A DAY: This doesn't mean that you should eat six full meals a day, but rather that you shouldn't let too much time pass without eating something. It can be an apple, a handful of nuts or a full meal, but try to eat regularly. The frequency will help fight hunger and maintain energy levels. Just make sure to stay within your daily caloric goal.

CONTROLLED INDULGENCE: We can derive great pleasure from food and it's okay to indulge. The key here is that you indulge on your terms. When you do stray from your normal routine, try to make sure that it's a planned and conscious decision rather than one made on impulse. Impulsive decisions tend to snowball, but if you made the decision ahead of time, there will be more satisfaction and less guilt after the fact, and you'll still be in control.

KEEPING A JOURNAL

A food journal is a great way to both assess your diet as well as a way to hold yourself accountable. Keeping a journal forces you to acknowledge your choices and, oftentimes, that's enough to stay on track. Try keeping a journal for a week to 10 days and then check to see how well you adhered to the rules.

When keeping the journal, make sure to enter things while you eat as it's easy to forget small details as the day goes on. Simply enter it into a notebook or go to www.RyanGeorgeFitness.com/doorframe, where I have a food journal template you can print and use. It's important to keep track of the food, the amount (calories) and the time. Alternatively, you can use an app to log your food. LiveStrong and MyFitnessPal are both great food-tracking apps.

COMMON FOOD MISCONCEPTIONS

THE MISCONCEPTION: Eating frequent meals will help boost your metabolism.

THE REALITY: Recent research suggests that there's no metabolic boost associated with eating frequently throughout the day.

THE MISCONCEPTION: Skipping breakfast and exercising first thing in the morning will help you burn more.

THE REALITY: While exercising on an empty stomach will utilize a higher percentage of fat for energy, that benefit is offset by the fact that you'll have less energy and will burn fewer total calories than if you eat breakfast.

THE MISCONCEPTION: Coffee is bad for you.

THE REALITY: Coffee can be very good for you—it's a great source of energy and can assist with post-exercise soreness. Plus, coffee contains powerful antioxidants and is associated with a decreased risk in many diseases. While coffee has its benefits, excessive consumption can still lead to dependence, restlessness and irritability, so use in moderation.

THE MISCONCEPTION: I need to consume 40-plus grams of protein per meal in order to put on muscle.

THE REALITY: We tend to place far too much emphasis on protein consumption, especially among those of us who are attempting to add muscle. Our bodies can only handle and process 15–20 grams of protein at a time. Protein shakes and bars are useful if you're having a hard time incorporating protein into your diet but, generally, you can get all of the protein that you need with a balanced and healthy diet.

THE MISCONCEPTION: I need to take a multivitamin supplement every day.

THE REALITY: Recent research seriously calls into question the effectiveness of multivitamin supplements. If you eat a balanced and healthy diet, you'll get all of the necessary vitamins and minerals straight from the source and won't have to worry about supplementation.

THE MISCONCEPTION: Sports drinks are ideal for exercise.

THE REALITY: While sports drinks can be useful in some situations, they're really little more than glorified sugar water. It's better to simply drink water and, if you need an extra shot of energy, add some honey.

THE MISCONCEPTION: A calorie is just a calorie.

THE REALITY: It's important to choose your calories wisely. A 2,000-calorie diet that's balanced and clean is far different from a 2,000-calorie diet that's high in saturated fats, sugar and processed foods. The kinds of calories you consume can have a significant impact on your hunger, insulin levels, energy levels, mood and digestion.

BEFORE YOU BEGIN

Before beginning an exercise program, it's important to be aware of the risks associated with exercise. Muscular and joint injuries are a risk with any exercise program. You can significantly minimize the risk by warming up properly, staying hydrated and progressing based on your fitness level. It's also important to exercise with proper form. If you have any joint injuries, speak with your doctor about what exercises you can and can't do.

In very rare instances, a person may develop heart problems that are induced by exercise. This happens for a variety of reasons. In some cases, it's genetic and in others it's a sign of coronary heart disease. Signs of heart trouble include dizziness, chest pain, light-headedness and vomiting. If you experience any of this, don't try to "work through it" — seek medical attention if the symptoms persist.

Obviously, the benefits of exercise far outweigh the risks, but it's important to check with your physician prior to beginning an exercise program to make sure that you're cleared to participate in a vigorous routine.

POSTURE

Posture is an important component in our quality of life, especially as we age. Poor posture can lead to muscle imbalances and eventually injuries. Poor posture can also be exacerbated by exercise, so you should assess and correct any posture problems as soon as possible.

If you have access to a full-length mirror, stand naturally in front of it and assess yourself from the ground up. Each point lists the ideal posture, or neutral position, followed by common problems:

FACING THE FRONT

FEET should be hip-width apart and pointing straight ahead. *Common problems:* One or both feet externally rotated; flat feet

KNEES should be lined up with the second and third toes. *Common problems:* Knock knees

HIPS should be level. *Common problems:* One side is higher than the other; rotation to one side

SHOULDERS should be level and shoulder blades retracted. *Common problems:* Protracted (rounded) shoulders; one or both shoulders elevated

HEAD should be neutral. *Common problems:* Tilted to the side

FACING THE SIDE

FEET should be neutral. *Common problems:* Inversion (sole rolls inward), eversion (sole rolls outward)

KNEES should be slightly bent. *Common problems:* Hyperextension

LOWER BACK should have a small curve. *Common problems:* Lordosis (extreme curvature); flat back

TRUNK should be neutral. *Common problems:* Kyphosis (rounded back); flat spine

SHOULDERS should be neutral. *Common problems:* Protraction, elevation

NECK should have a slight curve. *Common problems:* Forward extension

EARS, SHOULDERS, HIPS, KNEES AND ANKLES should all be in line.

EXERCISE POSITIONING

When exercising, it's necessary to maintain ideal posture as much as possible. Correct posture will make sure that your body is structurally sound and able to perform effectively. The following are the most common positions for exercises. *Standing upright:* Standing straight up in neutral position. *Standing bent over:* Sit back into a half-squat. Try to lower your torso as close to parallel to the floor as you can while maintaining a neutral spine. *Prone:* Lying with your abdomen facing the floor. *Supine:* Lying on your back. On a flat floor, your feet should be on the floor with your knees bent. There should be a small arch in your lower back. Your shoulder blades should be together and on the floor, while your head should be resting on the floor with your eyes facing straight up.

WARMING UP & COOLING DOWN

It's important to properly warm up prior to physical activity. Warming up will raise your body temperature, increase blood flow throughout your body and loosen up your joints. A proper warm-up will decrease your chances of injury during exercise. See page 185 for suggestions. A cool-down can also be a useful way to actively return your heart rate back to resting levels. Stretching should generally be done at the end of your workout and can serve as an effective means of cooling down. See page 189 for suggestions.

PART II
PROGRAMS

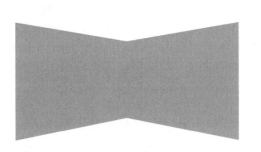

HOW TO USE THIS BOOK

In this section you'll find a variety of programs based on different goals and objectives. The first part covers fitness assessments that can be used to determine your fitness level as well as give you a baseline to measure your progress. The second part discusses a variety of programs and what they're good for, and also includes preset programs based on goals. This will give you the opportunity to understand how the programs function and the ability to design your own.

The information in this book will give you as much freedom as you'd like. If you like to design your programs, I'll provide you with the framework to do so. If you want every detail spelled out, there are fully fleshed-out programs for you to work with.

Programs are divided into beginner, intermediate and advanced workouts, giving you even more flexibility and the ability to progress from one level to the next. Exercise instructions appear in Part III; here are some explanations of terms I use.

- **Primary Muscles:** The muscles that do the most work in producing the movement. If you can, focus on these muscles when performing a particular exercise.

- **Secondary Muscles:** The muscles that assist in producing the movement.

- **Starting Position:** The position at which you begin your movement. Typically, a full repetition is completed every time you return to this position.

- **1, 2, 3, etc.:** The active part of the exercise. In some cases, there are multiple stages or movements.

- **Modification:** Ways to make the exercise easier.

- **Progression:** Ways to make the exercise harder.

Please note that I've included some very difficult exercises in this book. Many are progressions of other exercises, and you'll be asked to be comfortable with those prerequisite exercises before you try the advanced ones. Use caution when performing any of them; make sure that you've properly progressed up to these movements. As great as the exercises are, injury can result if you aren't safe.

FITNESS ASSESSMENTS

The fitness testing (assessments) is divided into two categories: baseline data and fitness testing. Fitness testing helps to serve three important purposes. First, it will give you a clear understanding of your fitness level, helping you identify potential strengths and weaknesses. You can then use this information to better plan and execute your exercise program. Second, fitness testing gives you a baseline with which to measure your progress. Using this baseline, you can create real and measurable goals. Regular reassessments will allow you to objectively measure your progress and make modifications if they're necessary. Finally, regular assessments serve as a form of accountability. Knowing that there's a reassessment coming up helps to keep you in check and provides motivation to maintain positive habits.

Testing should be conducted every four to eight weeks. You should allow enough time to make clear and measurable progress. Testing in very short intervals (one to two weeks) can be too short for noticeable progress. If the interval between testing periods is too long, you can run the risk of losing sight of your goals altogether. Since assessments give you the opportunity to modify a program that isn't working, waiting too long between them may cost you valuable time if your fitness program is not producing the results that you want.

USING THE ASSESSMENTS TO DETERMINE YOUR FITNESS LEVEL: Fitness level is not a one-size-fits-all situation. There are many aspects of fitness, such as overall strength, cardiovascular endurance and muscular endurance. Many of the tests below contain information on the norms for adults. You can use this information to determine your fitness strengths and weaknesses.

USING THE ASSESSMENTS TO SET GOALS: Each assessment gives you instructions on how to conduct the assessment. In addition, it contains information on goal setting. Use this information to create specific goals that can be measured the next time you conduct the assessments.

BASELINE DATA

These assessments are designed to measure your body's composition in a more detailed way than simply checking weight. These tests should be used to check your body's response to exercise. Baseline data tests should be performed at rest. The conditions under which you retest should be as close to identical as the initial testing as possible. Variables like time of day, clothing, food intake, caffeine intake, and scale can all skew the results if they vary from test to test. Ideally, the baseline data should be collected first thing in the morning before eating any food or drinking any caffeine. Record the data on the form on page 35.

WEIGHT: Use the same scale when assessing and reassessing; scales may be calibrated differently and can produce numbers that vary by as much as 5 pounds. *Goal setting:* If you want to lose weight, aim for no more than 2 pounds per week. Alternatively, if you're trying to gain weight, do not exceed 1–2 pounds per week.

BODY COMPOSITION (BODY FAT): This is the ratio of fat-free mass (muscle, bone, etc.) to fat weight in the body. Ideally, your fat weight should decrease and, depending on your goal, your fat-free mass should remain the same or increase. We measure body composition by body-fat percentage. For example, a 200-pound person with 20% body fat would have 40 pounds of fat weight. There are a few methods to determine body fat. If you have a scale that can determine it, make sure to reproduce the conditions whenever you reassess. Things like hydration levels, activity level and stress can all impact the results. If you have access to a gym or personal trainer, they may be able to use calipers to measure your body fat as well. In this case, make sure the same person performs the assessment every time.

FAT WEIGHT AND FAT-FREE MASS (FFM): Fat Weight = Bodyweight x Body Fat %, and Fat-Free Mass = Bodyweight–Fat. *Goal setting:* Your current goal will determine where your focus will lie. To increase definition, focus on the overall percentage. To build strength and/or muscle, focus on increasing FFM. A weight-loss goal will focus on a decrease in fat weight. If the focus is overall percentage, .5–1% per month is great.

RESTING HEART RATE (RHR): Your RHR is the number of times your heart beats per minute. As you become fitter, your RHR should lower. To measure it, find your pulse. There are three spots that you may use: temporal (on the temple), carotid (underneath the chin and on the front sides of your neck) and radial (on the thumb side of the wrist). Have a stopwatch or clock available. Gently palpate the area with your index and middle fingers. Once you find a pulse, count each beat for a full 60 seconds. *Goal setting:* Generally, a lower heart rate is a sign of more efficient cardiovascular function. For normal, healthy adults, it should fall between 60 and 100, according to the Mayo Clinic. If you're consistently above 100, consult with a physician. As a goal, you should try to be closer to the low end (60) than the higher end, and cardiovascular activity will help with that goal.

GIRTH MEASUREMENTS: Girth measurements are a good way to observe how your body is responding to exercise. Even if your weight remains the same, it's possible to lose inches around your body as your fitness level improves. These can be a bit of a challenge to measure, especially if you're by yourself. If possible, have a friend help you with this one. These tests are all done using a measuring tape, so make sure that the tape is parallel to the floor at all times and taut against the body.

• **Chest:** Place the tape under your arms and around your body at the nipple line.

• **Waist:** Use a mirror for this one—try to measure the narrowest part of your waist (between the rib cage and the navel).

• **Hips:** Stand with feet hip-width apart. Find your hip joint and measure around this point.

• **Abdomen:** Measure across your abdomen at the level of the navel.

• **Arms:** Measure the largest part of your upper arm. Measure each arm separately.

• **Thighs:** Measure the largest part of your upper thigh. Measure each leg separately.

• **Calves:** Measure the largest part of your calves. Make sure to measure each leg separately.

Goal setting: If your goal is to lose inches in an area, focus on losing about .5–1 inch at a time. If the goal is to increase inches in an area, focus on .25–.5 inch at a time.

BASELINE DATA FORM						
DATE						*GOAL*
WEIGHT						
BODY FAT %						
FAT WEIGHT						
FAT-FREE MASS						
RHR						
CHEST						
WAIST						
HIPS						
ABDOMEN						
ARMS (L/R)						
THIGHS (L/R)						
CALVES (L/R)						
OTHER						

FITNESS TESTING

Fitness testing consists of specific tests that measure your current fitness level in various categories. Make sure to be well rested and hydrated prior to these tests and that the area around you is clean, clear and safe prior to testing. Begin by warming up for 5 minutes and then proceed to the testing. If at any point you feel dizziness, nausea or joint pain, discontinue the test immediately.

Using the tables with each test, you can determine your fitness level in a number of categories. You can use this information to build on your strengths and improve on any weaknesses. Record your data in the form below. While it's not necessary to perform all of the tests and record all of your measurements, the more data that you record, the more complete and accurate your fitness profile will be.

FITNESS TESTING MEASUREMENTS						
DATE						GOAL
PULL-UP						
PUSH-UP						
CHAIR SQUAT						
AB CURL						
PLANK						
1.5 MILES						
1-MINUTE SQUAT THRUST						

PULL-UP: This is a test for upper-body strength. Do a standard pull-up (page 98). Terminate the test when you can't perform a full pull-up without good form. If you can't perform one full pull-up, then you may modify the movement by performing a band-assisted pull-up (page 119) or chair-assisted pull-up (page 118) or shortening the ROM. *Goal setting:* Try to increase 1 repetition every 1 to 2 weeks. To determine the program level you should start with, follow these guidelines:

- If you can't complete 1 pull-up but you can complete the modified versions listed above, begin the Level 1 pull-up development program (page 90).
- If you can only complete 1 pull-up, begin the Level 2 pull-up development program (page 90).
- If you can complete 2–3 pull-ups, begin the Level 3 pull-up development program (page 91).

PULL-UP TEST*		
	MALE	*FEMALE*
EXCELLENT	> 13	> 6
ABOVE AVERAGE	9–13	5–6
AVERAGE	6–8	3–4
BELOW AVERAGE	3–5	1–2
POOR	< 3	0

* Testing guidelines based on U.S. Marines testing criteria.

PUSH-UP: This is a test for upper-body strength and endurance. Follow the form for push-ups on page 139. Terminate the test when you can't complete another repetition with good form. Count the total number of repetitions without rest. If you can't perform 1 full push-up, you may perform modified push-ups by dropping your knees to the floor. *Goal setting:* Try to increase 1 to 2 repetitions per week.

PUSH-UP TEST*					
MEN (AGE)	*20–29*	*30–39*	*40–49*	*50–59*	*60+*
EXCELLENT	54+	44+	39+	34+	29+
ABOVE AVERAGE	45–54	35–44	30–39	25–34	20–29
AVERAGE	35–44	24–34	20–29	15–24	10–19
BELOW AVERAGE	20–34	15–24	12–19	8–14	5–9
POOR	19 or fewer	14 or fewer	11 or fewer	7 or fewer	4 or fewer
WOMEN (AGE)	*20–29*	*30–39*	*40–49*	*50–59*	*60+*
EXCELLENT	48+	39+	34+	29+	19+
ABOVE AVERAGE	34–48	25–39	20–34	15–29	15–19
AVERAGE	17–33	12–24	8–19	6–14	3–4
BELOW AVERAGE	6–16	4–11	3–7	2–5	1–2
POOR	5 or fewer	3 or fewer	2 or fewer	1 or fewer	none

* Test based on the World Instructor Training Schools (WITS) testing criteria.

CHAIR SQUAT: This is a test for lower-body endurance. Set up a chair, bench or box that leaves your knees bent about 90 degrees when you're sitting. Stand up with the chair behind you. Use the form for a squat on page 146 until your bottom lightly touches the chair. Immediately stand back up. Terminate the test when you can't complete another repetition with good form. Count the number of consecutive repetitions without a break. *Goal setting:* Try to increase 1 repetition per week.

CHAIR SQUAT TEST*					
MEN (AGE)	20–29	30–39	40–49	50–59	60+
EXCELLENT	34+	32+	29+	26+	23+
ABOVE AVERAGE	30–32	27–29	24–26	21–23	18–20
AVERAGE	27–29	24–26	21–23	18–20	15–17
BELOW AVERAGE	24–26	21–23	18–20	15–17	12–14
POOR	23 or fewer	20 or fewer	17 or fewer	14 or fewer	11 or fewer
WOMEN (AGE)	20–29	30–39	40–49	50–59	60+
EXCELLENT	29+	26+	23+	20+	17+
ABOVE AVERAGE	24–16	21–23	18–20	15–17	12–14
AVERAGE	21–23	18–20	15–17	12–14	9–11
BELOW AVERAGE	18–20	15–17	12–14	9–11	6–8
POOR	17 or fewer	14 or fewer	11 or fewer	8 or fewer	6 or fewer

* Test based on the American College of Sports Medicine (ACSM) testing criteria.

ABDOMINAL CURL-UP: This is a test for abdominal endurance. Use the form for a crunch on page 165. Terminate when you can't complete another repetition with good form. Count the number of consecutive repetitions without a break. *Goal setting:* Try to increase 1 repetition per week.

ABDOMINAL CRUNCH TEST*					
MEN (AGE)	20–29	30–39	40–49	50–59	60+
EXCELLENT	65	60	50	40	30
ABOVE AVERAGE	50	45	40	25	n/a
AVERAGE	35	30	25	15	9
BELOW AVERAGE	20	15	10	5	n/a
POOR	19 or fewer	14 or fewer	9 or fewer	4 or fewer	3 or fewer
WOMEN (AGE)	20–29	30–39	40–49	50–59	60+
EXCELLENT	55	50	40	30	n/a
ABOVE AVERAGE	45	40	25	15	10
AVERAGE	33	25	15	10	n/a
BELOW AVERAGE	13	10	6	4	3
POOR	12 or fewer	9 or fewer	5 or fewer	3 or fewer	n/a

* Test based on the American College of Sports Medicine (ACSM) testing criteria.

PLANK: This is a test for core stability and endurance. Use the form for a plank on page 161. Using a timer, count how many seconds you can hold the plank. Terminate when you can no longer hold the correct position or if you feel pain in your lower back. Thirty seconds is average and anything more than 1 minute is great. Make sure to maintain proper form throughout. *Goal setting:* Try to increase by 5 seconds every week until you reach 1 minute. It's not necessary to exceed 1 minute.

1.5-MILE WALK/RUN: This is a test for aerobic endurance. It's used to estimate your VO2 max, which represents your body's ability to extract oxygen from the blood. The goal is to complete this test in minimal time, so have a timer available. Upon beginning, start the timer and run. Stop the timer when you reach 1.5 miles and record it. If you can't complete 1.5 miles, record both the distance and the time.

This is an intense test so, if you're not used to this kind of activity, it may be helpful to do a trial run prior to the actual test. Use the chart below to determine your level. *Goal setting:* A great goal would be to improve your time by 1 minute the next time you test.

1.5-MILE TEST*					
MALE	*20–29*	*30–39*	*40–49*	*50–59*	*60+*
EXCELLENT	10:08	10:38	11:09	12:08	13:25
ABOVE AVERAGE	11:27	12:01	12:43	13:18	15:01
AVERAGE	11:58	12:25	13:05	14:33	16:19
BELOW AVERAGE	13:08	13:48	14:33	16:16	18:39
POOR	15:14	15:56	17:04	19:24	23:27
WOMEN	*19–29*	*30–39*	*40–49*	*50–59*	*60+*
EXCELLENT	11:56	12:53	13:38	15:14	16:46
ABOVE AVERAGE	13:25	14:33	15:17	17:19	18:52
AVERAGE	14:15	15:14	16:13	18:05	20:08
BELOW AVERAGE	15:56	16:46	18:26	20:17	22:34
POOR	18:39	20:13	21:52	23:55	26:32

* Test based on the World Instructor Training Schools (WITS) testing criteria.

1-MINUTE SQUAT THRUST: This is a test for anaerobic endurance. Use the form for squat thrusts on page 183. Set a timer for 1 minute. Begin the timer and complete as many as you can in 1 minute. Record the number. *Goal setting:* Try to increase by 1 repetition every 1 to 2 weeks.

GOAL SETTING

Goal setting is an important part of maintaining a fitness program. While it helps to set goals at the beginning of your program, keep in mind that goals are also variable and can easily change over time. You may begin an exercise program simply to get in shape and then decide that you want to run a marathon. Alternatively, a person may begin a high-intensity program only to find out that they're pregnant.

Goal setting is divided into three sections: immediate, short- and long-term goals. *Immediate goals* typically represent things that you plan on implementing immediately, like eliminating soda or increasing your exercise intensity. These tend to represent changes in habits. *Short-term goals* represent your goals in between assessments. These goals are set for four to eight weeks at a time. Here you'll focus on the measurements and fitness tests. While you don't necessarily have to set a goal for every test, you should choose something appropriate to your objective. Every time you assess and reassess, try to set goals for the next assessment. *Long-term goals* are your ultimate goals or objectives. Your short-term goals should be consistently building toward these goals. Your long-term goals are personal and may be numbers based (lose 30 pounds), objective based (compete in a triathlon) or functional (walk up stairs without shortness of breath). When beginning an exercise program, create a milestone checklist for your long-term goals. Reward yourself whenever you achieve one and create a new goal to replace it.

MILESTONE CHECKLIST			
MILESTONE	*DESCRIBE GOAL*	*GOAL DATE*	*DATE COMPLETED*

PROGRAMMING YOUR FITNESS GOALS		
PROGRAM	**FOCUS**	**SHORT-TERM GOALS**
GENERAL FITNESS	Overall health and well-being.	• Reduce body fat percentage • Reduce inches on the waist and abdomen • Increase push-ups and pull-ups • Reduce time on 1.5-mile run
WEIGHT LOSS	Decrease in total bodyweight; endurance is an important component.	• Reduce fat weight • Reduce inches on the waist and abdomen • Reduce overall weight • Reduce time on 1.5-mile run
INCREASED MUSCULAR STRENGTH	Increase in muscle mass and improved performance of strength movements.	• Increase fat-free mass • Increase pull-ups and push-ups • Increase inches in the chest, arms and thighs • Reduce body fat percentage
BODY SCULPTING	Combination of increased fat-free mass and decreased body fat. Ideally an increase in muscular size will also occur. A clean diet is especially important with this goal.	• Reduce body fat percentage • Increase fat-free mass • Decrease inches in the waist, abdomen and hips • Decrease fat weight • Increase inches in the chest, arms and thighs
CARDIO CONDITIONING	Improve VO2 max and aerobic capacity.	• Reduce time on 1.5-mile run • Increase number of 1-minute squat thrust • Reduce body fat percentage
ATHLETIC CONDITIONING	Improve both overall strength and aerobic capacity.	• Reduce time on 1.5-mile run • Increase number of 1-minute squat thrust • Reduce body fat percentage • Decrease fat weight • Increase total push-ups, crunches and squats • Increase fat-free mass

PROGRAM DESIGN

The process of developing a fitness program involves adhering to certain set principles. Knowing how to apply these principles to your fitness program is a major key to success. Whether you fit into the general or performance-based categories, these principles apply across the board and need to be used in any program in order to be as effective as possible.

SPECIFICITY: The specificity principle says that your body will adapt specifically to the kind of exercise that you participate in. The more specific the goal or skill, the more specific the training needs to be. A marathon runner, for example, needs a high level of aerobic endurance. Activities like long-distance running, cycling and swimming are all beneficial since they help develop aerobic endurance. Heavy weight training, on the other hand, wouldn't translate as well because it doesn't focus on aerobic endurance.

Application: When developing an exercise program, it's important to determine what your goals are. Once you've you set your objectives, you can determine the best approach. A general fitness program offers more flexibility, whereas a more sport- or movement-specific program will require more specificity.

CONSISTENCY: For most people, consistency is the single most important factor in determining the success of a fitness program. While the body is great at adapting to stress, the opposite is also true. Commonly referred to as the "use it or lose it" principle, the body will regress if you don't provide it with sufficient stress in the form of exercise. All it takes is 10 days for muscles to atrophy and to lose a significant amount of your aerobic capacity.

Consistency is also important because, ideally, exercise should be a part of your lifestyle. Most people aren't passionate about exercise, so it's important to find a routine that's manageable but consistent in order to make it a regular thing. It's easy to make excuses and skip training. I've witnessed time and time again how an inconsistent regimen can quickly turn into an extended absence from exercise. Over time, a consistent program should ingrain itself into your life.

Application: When developing an exercise program, it's important to work out a routine that's manageable both physically and psychologically. Find times that are convenient and a routine that you can keep up for the foreseeable future.

EFFICIENCY: When it comes to improving your fitness, in most situations you should emphasize quality over quantity. It's important to maximize your time exercising. Using programs like high-intensity interval training (HIIT), you can get more work done in a 20-minute workout than you can in an hour of traditional training. This helps to eliminate time as an obstacle. The key is to work as hard as you can with minimal rest over a short period of time.

Application: When developing an exercise program, focus on the intensity and volume of work rather than the amount of time you spend working out. If you work hard enough, two high-intensity 20-minute sessions a week can be more effective than five moderate-intensity one-hour sessions.

PROGRESSION: As I mentioned earlier, we benefit from exercise because our body has to adapt to new stress and stimuli. If we don't introduce new stress, the body has no need to adapt and therefore will maintain its fitness level or regress. This is often the cause of the dreaded "plateau." The principle of progression, or progressive overload, says that we must constantly and consistently push ourselves beyond what our bodies are used to in order to progress.

Application: When designing an exercise program, it's important to improve some variable every few weeks in order to make progress. If you begin a program being able to complete 5 pull-ups, then your goal should be to increase that number over time. If three months pass and you're still performing 5 pull-ups at a time, then you're maintaining the status quo but will not derive any increase in strength or endurance from that exercise.

REST AND RECOVERY: Rest and recovery are very commonly overlooked when developing an exercise program. When you exercise, you place stress on the body, breaking it down a little. While resting, your body adapts by building back stronger. If you don't allow yourself time to recover, exercise starts to follow the law of diminishing returns. Your body rebuilds itself while at rest. Too little rest can lead to overtraining, which can then lead to physical regression and injuries. Optimal rest time varies based on your current fitness level as well as the activity, but most people should have at least two rest days per week.

Application: When designing a strength-training program, keep in mind that you should leave 24–48 hours between training body parts. If you're working on your chest on Monday, for example, you wouldn't want to work your chest again until Wednesday or Thursday.

OTHER IMPORTANT FITNESS CONCEPTS

In addition to the primary fitness principles, there are other important concepts to understand when developing a fitness program.

PLATEAU: Sometimes we reach a point in an exercise program where, no matter how much we try, we can't seem to make any progress. This is often referred to as a plateau and is usually a sign that we need to change things up.

PERIODIZATION: Periodization is a method of changing a fitness program in set intervals. Usually, each cycle has its own set of specific goals. This is a great way to fight a plateau as you never stick with one training method for too long. To give an example, if your ultimate goal is to both add 10 pounds of muscle and lose 10 pounds of fat, a periodized program would be the most efficient. The two goals conflict quite a bit since it would be difficult to both add 10 pounds of muscle and lose 10 pounds of fat using the same program. With a periodized program, you'd spend 8–12 weeks focused only on muscle building. Once you've added the 10 pounds of muscle, you'd focus on fat loss.

OVERTRAINING: Overtraining happens when a person gets too much exercise, too little rest or a combination of the two. When designing an exercise program, it's important to consider your current condition. While progression is important, it should be gradual. Signs of overtraining include increased injuries, constant soreness, unusual fatigue and irritability.

PROGRAMMING FAQS

A few questions pop up regularly when developing and implementing a fitness program. I answer the most important questions below.

Q: What should I do if I can't perform pull-ups?

A: Substitute one of these three modifications and incorporate the pull-up development program (page 90) into your fitness routine in order to progress to full pull-ups: Short-Range Pull-Up (pages 116 and 117), Band-Assisted Pull-Up (page 119), Chair-Assisted Pull-Up (page 118).

Q: What should I do if I can't perform an exercise?

A: The exercise will typically include directions on how to modify it. If not, one common way is to perform the movement with a shorter ROM. As you progress with the program, try to incrementally increase the ROM in order to eventually reach the full ROM.

Q: What should I do if an exercise is too easy?

A: You have a couple of options. If the exercise includes ways to progress that specific exercise, go ahead and try that. Another option is to adjust one of the variables (discussed on page 12).

Q: What if I can't complete the set number of repetitions?

A: Complete as many as you can with good form and then modify the movement if possible. For example, if you have a set of 10 pull-ups and you can only complete 7, after the seventh pull-up, modify the movement by switching to short ROM pull-ups for the final three. The same applies if the exercise is for time. If you have to complete as many hanging leg curls as possible in 30 seconds, modify the movement if you reach a point where you can't perform full ROM hanging leg curls.

Q: Which program can I use?

A: When choosing among the programs, first consider your goal. Once you have your goal, the programs are broken up into beginner, intermediate and advanced levels. A beginner program is for anyone. Check the prerequisites for the intermediate and advanced programs, as they'll include some basic requirements based on your assessment results and exercise history.

Q: What does "#" mean?

A: Some of the exercises included in your program will be based on your assessment results. If the repetition box has a "#," that means you have to input your most recent assessment number.

Q: If an exercise uses one arm, leg or side at a time, how should I read the sets/reps?

A: Sets and reps apply to each side separately. For example, if a program shows 3 sets of 10 reps for a single-leg squat, perform 3 sets of 10 repetitions on each leg, or 20 combined. Unless it's specified, you may perform them either consecutively or alternately.

TEMPLATES

If you're designing your own workout, this section will guide you through the process of selecting the correct program. Selecting the right program is straightforward (see "Goal Setting" on page 40). First, determine your primary goal and then select a program that focuses on that goal. Once you've selected a program, the next step is to determine your exercises. It's best to select a variety of exercises that, together, cover all of the muscle groups throughout the body. This will help to protect against muscle imbalances. Tempo and rest are both determined based on your goal. Muscle-building programs typically require a slower tempo and longer rest, while cardio and conditioning programs require a faster tempo and shorter rest.

Each program is designed to follow over six weeks. Once you've completed the six weeks, you may redo the same workout or try out another template. If after six weeks the workout is still difficult, it may be best to stick with it for another six weeks. If you want something more challenging or your goals change, switch to a different template. For blank templates (single sets, supersets, trisets, timed circuit, repetition circuit, tabatas and modified tabatas) for customizing your own program, go to www.RyanGeorgeFitness.com/doorframe.

SINGLE SET SAMPLE TEMPLATE

GOOD FOR: General fitness, strength building

With single sets, you perform all of the required sets for each exercise before moving on to the next. Using the example below for week 1, you'd perform 3 sets of 10 reps (3x10) of push-ups, with 60 seconds of rest in between each set. Move on to press-ups after you finish with your third set of push-ups. Also be aware of the tempo. While the push-up has a normal tempo, the press-up is a slower negative portion and the plank is an isometric hold.

	SINGLE SET	WEEK 1 set x rep	WEEK 2 set x rep	WEEK 3 set x rep	WEEK 4 set x rep	WEEK 5 set x rep	WEEK 6 set x rep
DAY 1	**PUSH-UP** *tempo:* 1-1-3 | *rest:* 60 sec	3x10	3x10	3x12	3x15	3x20	3x20
	PRESS-UP *tempo:* 1-1-2 | *rest:* 60 sec	3x8	3x8	3x10	3x12	3x12	3x12
	PLANK *tempo:* 1-30-1 | *rest:* 60 sec	2x1	2x1	2x1	3x1	3x1	3x1

SUPERSETS SAMPLE TEMPLATE

GOOD FOR: Time efficient, general fitness, muscular endurance

Supersets combine two exercises that are performed back to back with little to no rest. Sets are performed in pairs and can be designed to work opposing muscle groups (e.g., biceps/triceps), upper body and lower body, or the same muscle group. In week 1 of the example below, you'd perform alternate-grip pull-ups (exercise 1a), rest 15 seconds and perform squats (exercise 1b), followed by another 30-second rest period. You'd then repeat for your second and third sets. After your third set, you'd begin doing push-ups (exercise 2a), immediately followed by split squats (exercise 2b) since there's no rest period for this pair.

	SUPERSETS	WEEK 1 set x rep	WEEK 2 set x rep	WEEK 3 set x rep	WEEK 4 set x rep	WEEK 5 set x rep	WEEK 6 set x rep
DAY 1	**1a. ALTERNATE-GRIP PULL-UP** *tempo:* 1-1-5 | *rest:* 15 sec	3x4	3x4	3x5	3x5	3x6	3x6
	1b. SQUAT *tempo:* 1-1-5 | *rest:* 30 sec	3x12	3x12	3x12	3x12	3x12	3x12
	2a. PUSH-UP *tempo:* 1-1-5 | *rest:* 0 sec	3x12	3x12	3x12	3x12	3x12	3x12
	2b. SPLIT SQUAT *tempo:* 1-1-5 | *rest:* 30 sec	3x6	3x7	3x8	3x8	3x9	3x9

TRISETS SAMPLE TEMPLATE

GOOD FOR: Time efficient, total body, general fitness, conditioning, weight loss

Trisets follow the same rules as supersets except that you're performing three exercises at a time. Exercises can be chosen among upper, lower, abdominal and cardio conditioning.

	TRISETS	WEEK 1 set x rep	WEEK 2 set x rep	WEEK 3 set x rep	WEEK 4 set x rep	WEEK 5 set x rep	WEEK 6 set x rep
DAY 1	**1a. CHIN-UP** *tempo:* 1-1-3 | *rest:* 10 sec	3x10	3x10	3x10	3x11	3x11	3x12
	1b. SQUAT *tempo:* 1-1-3 | *rest:* 10 sec	3x20	3x20	3x20	3x20	3x20	3x20
	1c. TOTAL-BODY CRUNCH *tempo:* 1-1-2 | *rest:* 130 sec	3x12	3x12	3x12	3x15	3x15	3x15

TIMED CIRCUIT SAMPLE TEMPLATE

GOOD FOR: Weight loss, cardio conditioning, muscle endurance

Circuit training is a way to increase your heart rate by performing a series of exercises with little to no rest in between. In the example below, you'd perform single-leg bridge for 30 seconds, followed by a 30-second rest. You'd then move on to plank for 30 seconds, followed by a 30-second rest. Timed circuits emphasize speed of movement so there's no specified tempo. If you want to increase the difficulty, increase the speed (while maintaining proper form); if you want to decrease the difficulty, decrease the speed. In this routine, you'd repeat the full circuit two additional times as indicated by the rounds at the bottom.

	TIMED CIRCUIT	WEEK 1 duration	WEEK 2 duration	WEEK 3 duration	WEEK 4 duration	WEEK 5 duration	WEEK 6 duration
DAY 1	**SINGLE-LEG BRIDGE** rest: 30 sec	30 sec	30 sec	35 sec	35 sec	40 sec	40 sec
	PLANK rest: 30 sec	30 sec	30 sec	35 sec	35 sec	40 sec	40 sec
	SPEED SQUAT rest: 30 sec	30 sec	30 sec	35 sec	35 sec	40 sec	40 sec
	DIP WITH BAR rest: 30 sec	30 sec	30 sec	35 sec	35 sec	40 sec	40 sec
	ROUNDS	2	3	2	3	2	3

REPETITION CIRCUIT SAMPLE TEMPLATE

GOOD FOR: Weight loss, cardio conditioning, muscle endurance, strength

The repetition circuit works the same as the timed circuit with the exception that you're completing a specified number of repetitions instead of doing so for time. In this routine, you'd repeat the full circuit two additional times as indicated by the rounds at the bottom.

	REPETITION CIRCUIT	WEEK 1 reps	WEEK 2 reps	WEEK 3 reps	WEEK 4 reps	WEEK 5 reps	WEEK 6 reps
DAY 1	**STANDARD PULL-UP** tempo: 1-1-3 | rest: 15 sec	10	10	12	12	15	15
	STAGGERED PULL-UP tempo: 1-1-3 | rest: 15 sec	10	10	12	12	15	15
	HANGING LEG RAISE tempo: 1-1-2 | rest: 15 sec	10	10	12	12	15	15
	ROUNDS	3	3	3	3	3	3

TABATA SAMPLE TEMPLATE

GOOD FOR: Cardio conditioning, muscle endurance, athletic conditioning, strength

Each exercise in a tabata consists of eight 20-second rounds broken up with 10-second rest periods. During the working periods, move as quickly as you can. The objective is to maximize your intensity and use the rest periods to recover enough to begin again. Find a speed that works for you—if anything is too difficult, slow down; if it's easy, speed up.

Using the example below, perform squat jumps for 20 seconds, followed by a 10-second rest. Immediately after the 10-second rest, begin your second 20-second round, followed by another 10-second rest. Continue this way until you've completed four total 20-second rounds of squat jumps before you move on to push-ups.

	TABATA	WEEK 1 sets x duration	WEEK 2 sets x duration	WEEK 3 sets x duration	WEEK 4 sets x duration	WEEK 5 sets x duration	WEEK 6 sets x duration
DAY 1	**SQUAT JUMP** *rest:* 10 sec between rounds	4x20 sec	4x20 sec	4x20 sec	4x20 sec	4x20 sec	4x20 sec
	PUSH-UP *rest:* 10 sec between rounds	4x20 sec	4x20 sec	4x20 sec	4x20 sec	4x20 sec	4x20 sec

MODIFIED TABATA SAMPLE TEMPLATE

GOOD FOR: Cardio conditioning, muscle endurance, athletic conditioning, strength

Modified tabatas follow the same rules as tabatas except that you alternate between two exercises. Using the example below, perform exercise 1a (high knees) for 20 seconds, followed by a 10-second rest. Immediately following the rest, begin exercise 1b (high twist) for 20 seconds, followed by a 10-second rest. Continue this way until you've completed eight total rounds (four of each exercise). Then proceed to the next pair of exercises in the chart.

	MODIFIED TABATA	WEEK 1 sets x duration	WEEK 2 sets x duration	WEEK 3 sets x duration	WEEK 4 sets x duration	WEEK 5 sets x duration	WEEK 6 sets x duration
DAY 1	**1a. HIGH KNEES** *rest:* 10 sec between rounds	4x20 sec	4x20 sec	4x20 sec	4x20 sec	4x20 sec	4x20 sec
	1b. HIGH TWIST *rest:* 10 sec between rounds	4x20 sec	4x20 sec	4x20 sec	4x20 sec	4x20 sec	4x20 sec
	2a. SKATER *rest:* 10 sec between rounds	4x20 sec	4x20 sec	4x20 sec	4x20 sec	4x20 sec	4x20 sec
	2b. PRESS-UP *rest:* 10 sec between rounds	4x20 sec	4x20 sec	4x20 sec	4x20 sec	4x20 sec	4x20 sec

PROGRAMS

These preset fitness programs are designed around a specific goal and contain all of the information you need to begin working out. The programs are designed using a periodized format. Periodization is an efficient way to achieve fitness goals; it allows you to focus on different objectives, which over time will help you quickly achieve your overall goal.

Each program is designed to follow over six weeks. Once you've completed the six weeks, you may redo the same workout or try out another. If after six weeks the workout is still difficult, it may be best to stick with it for another six weeks. If you want something more challenging or your goals change, you should switch to a different program.

Imagine that your goal is to both put on significant muscle and lose significant fat. These are two separate and distinct goals. It would be difficult to achieve both at the same time because the methods of training are completely counter to each other. In order to efficiently reach this goal, you may spend a six-week period focused only on building muscle. You can then follow that up with a six-week period where your focus is cardio conditioning so you begin to drop some weight and improve your aerobic capacity. You can then spend the next six weeks focused only on weight loss. In this way, you'll have the extra muscle and aerobic capacity so when you begin the real weight-loss phase, you'll be in a great position to achieve your ultimate goal of building muscle and losing weight.

These preset programs are all designed with this in mind. The programs are arranged based on the ultimate goal, or macrocycle. Each macrocycle covers 18 weeks but can be modified by adding or subtracting weeks from the different mesocycles. Each macrocycle consists of three six-week mesocycles, which focus on three different objectives. Like the macrocycles, the mesocycles can also be modified. When you're finished with a full macrocycle, you can repeat, advance to another or design your own program.

Most programs will show 3 days a week. This doesn't mean that you're limited to 3 days. Simply repeat days 1, 2 and 3 in that order to work out 4, 5 or 6 days a week. You should work out a minimum of 3 days, with 4 to 5 days being ideal.

CHOOSING THE CORRECT PROGRAM & LEVEL: The first step to choosing the correct program is determining your overall goal or objective. Once you've decided on this, select the program that matches that goal. The second step is determining which level to begin with. Beginner programs are appropriate for anyone and are especially good to start with if you aren't currently exercising regularly. Intermediate and advanced programs have prerequisites, which consist of a combination of fitness-assessment results and the completion of other fitness programs. If you meet the prerequisites for any program, you can begin that program. If you don't, complete one of the beginner programs before advancing to the intermediate and advanced programs. For some preset advanced programs for general fitness, weight loss and body sculpting, go to www.RyanGeorgeFitness.com/doorframe.

GENERAL FITNESS (BEGINNER)

PREREQUISITE: There are no prerequisites for the beginner program.

MACROCYCLE: *Two six-week mesocycles:* Single Set, Superset. *Extras:* cardio 2–3 days/week.

	SINGLE SET	*WEEK 1* *set x rep*	*WEEK 2* *set x rep*	*WEEK 3* *set x rep*	*WEEK 4* *set x rep*	*WEEK 5* *set x rep*	*WEEK 6* *set x rep*
DAY 1	***CHIN-UP*** *tempo:* 1-1-3 | *rest:* 90 sec	2x5	2x5	3x6	3x6	3x7	3x7
	PUSH-UP *tempo:* 1-1-3 | *rest:* 60	2x#	2x#	3x#+1	3x#+1	3x#+2	3x#+3
	DIP WITH BAR *tempo:* 1-1-3 | rest 60 sec	2x8	2x8	3x9	3x9	3x10	3x12
	STANDARD PULL-UP *tempo:* 1-1-3 | *rest:* 90 sec	2x#	2x#	3x#+1	3x#+1	3x#+2	3x#+3
	PLANK WALK-UP *tempo:* 1-1-2 | *rest:* 30 sec	2x8	2x8	3x9	3x9	3x10	3x11
	DIAMOND PUSH-UP tempo:1-1-2 | rest: 60 sec	2x8	2x8	3x9	3x9	3x10	3x10
	STANDING WALK-OUT tempo:1-1-3 | rest: 45 sec	2x8	2x8	3x10	3x10	3x12	3x12
	PARALLEL GRIP PULL-UP tempo:1-1-3 | *rest:* 90 sec	2x5	2x5	3x6	3x6	3x7	3x7
DAY 2	***SQUAT*** *tempo:* 1-1-3 | *rest:* 30 sec	2x15	2x15	3x20	3x20	3x20	3x25
	FORWARD LUNGE *tempo:* 1-1-3 | rest: 45 sec	2x8	2x8	3x10	3x10	3x12	3x12
	CALF RAISE *tempo:* 1-1-2 | *rest:* 30 sec	2x10	2x10	3x12	3x12	3x15	3x15
	SINGLE-LEG BRIDGE *tempo:* 1-1-2 | *rest:* 30 sec	2x8	2x8	3x10	3x10	3x12	3x12
	CORE WALK-OUT *tempo:* 1-1-5 | *rest:* 45 sec	2x8	2x8	3x10	3x10	3x12	3x12
	PLANK *tempo:* 1-30-1 | *rest:* 30 sec	2x1	2x1	2x1	2x1	2x1	2x1
	SIDE PLANK *tempo:* 1-1-2 | *rest:* 45 sec	2x8	2x8	3x10	3x10	3x12	3x12
	STRAIGHT-LEG RAISE *tempo:* 1-1-3 | *rest:* 60 sec	2x6	2x6	2x6	3x8	3x8	3x10

Exercise						
SIDE-FACING PULL-UP *tempo:* 1-1-3 | *rest:* 60 sec	2x3 (ea)	2x3 (ea)	3x4 (ea)	3x4 (ea)	3x5 (ea)	3x5 (ea)
CHAIR DIP *tempo:* 1-1-2 | *rest:* 60 sec	2x8	2x8	3x10	3x10	3x12	3x12
ALTERNATE-GRIP PULL-UP *tempo:* 1-1-3 | *rest:* 60 sec	2x3 (ea)	2x3 (ea)	3x4 (ea)	3x4 (ea)	3x5 (ea)	3x5 (ea)
PUSH-UP WITH BAR *tempo:* 1-1-3 | *rest:* 60 sec	2x#	2x#	3x#+1	3x#+1	3x#+3	3x#+4
CRUNCH *tempo:* 1-1-1 | *rest:* 60 sec	2x20	2x20	3x25	3x25	3x25	3x25
LEG CURL *tempo:* 1-1-3 | *rest:* 45 sec	2x8	2x8	3x10	3x10	3x10	3x10
BICYCLE CRUNCH *tempo:* 1-1-1 | *rest:* 45 sec	2x8	2x8	3x10	3x10	3x12	3x15
HANGING LEG CURL *tempo:* 1-1-3 | *rest:* 45 sec	2x8	2x8	3x10	3x10	3x10	3x10

SUPERSETS	WEEK 1 *set x rep*	WEEK 2 *set x rep*	WEEK 3 *set x rep*	WEEK 4 *set x rep*	WEEK 5 *set x rep*	WEEK 6 *set x rep*
1a. CHIN-UP *tempo:* 1-1-3 | *rest:* 10 sec	3x7	3x7	3x7	3x8	3x8	3x8
1b. CRUNCH *tempo:* 1-1-1 | *rest:* 30 sec	3x25	3x25	3x30	3x30	3x30	3x35
2a. PUSH-UP *tempo:* 1-1-3 | *rest:* 10 sec	3x#+1	3x#+1	3x#+2	3x#+2	3x#+3	3x#+4
2b. TOTAL-BODY CRUNCH *tempo:* 1-1-2 | *rest:* 30 sec	3x8	3x10	3x10	3x12	3x12	3x15
3a. DIP WITH BAR *tempo:* 1-1-2 | *rest:* 10 sec	3x8	3x8	3x10	3x10	3x12	3x12
3b. HANGING LEG CURL *tempo:* 1-1-3 | *rest:* 30 sec	3x10	3x10	3x12	3x12	3x12	3x12
4a. PULL-UP *tempo:* 1-1-3 | *rest:* 10 sec	3x#	3x#+1	3x#+1	3x#+2	3x#+2	3x#+3
4b. BICYCLE CRUNCH *tempo:* 1-1-1 | *rest:* 30 sec	3x12	3x12	3x15	3x15	3x15	3x15
5a. ALTERNATE-GRIP PULL-UP *tempo:* 1-1-3 | *rest:* 10 sec	3x4 (ea)	3x4 (ea)	3x5 (ea)	3x5 (ea)	3x6 (ea)	3x6 (ea)
5b. LEG CURL *tempo:* 1-1-2 | *rest:* 30 sec	3x10	3x10	3x12	3x12	3x15	3x15

	Exercise						
DAY 2	**1a. SQUAT** *tempo:* 1-1-3 | *rest:* 10 sec	3x15	3x15	3x15	3x20	3x20	3x20
	1b. PLANK *tempo:* 1-45-1 | *rest:* 30 sec	3x1	3x1	3x1	3x1	3x1	3x1
	2a. FORWARD LUNGE *tempo:* 1-1-3 | *rest:* 10 sec	3x10	3x12	3x12	3x12	3x15	3x15
	2b. CORE WALK-OUT *tempo:* 1-1-3 | *rest:* 30 sec	3x10	3x10	3x10	3x12	3x12	3x12
	3a. CALF RAISE *tempo:* 1-1-2 | *rest:* 10 sec	3x12	3x12	3x12	3x15	3x15	3x20
	3b. STRAIGHT-LEG RAISE *tempo:* 1-1-3 | *rest:* 30 sec	3x10	3x10	3x12	3x12	3x12	3x12
	4a. SPLIT SQUAT *tempo:* 1-1-3 | *rest:* 10 sec	3x10	3x10	3x10	3x10	3x12	3x12
	4b. PLANK WITH ARM EXTENSION *tempo:* 1-1-1 | *rest:* 30 sec	3x12	3x12	3x12	3x15	3x15	3x15
	5a. SINGLE-LEG BRIDGE *tempo:* 1-1-2 | *rest:* 10 sec	3x12	3x12	3x12	3x15	3x15	3x15
	5b. SIDE PLANK *tempo:* 1-1-2 | *rest:* 30 sec	3x1	3x1	3x1	3x1	3x1	3x1
DAY 3	**1a. CHAIR DIP** *tempo:* 1-1-2 | *rest:* 10 sec	3x10	3x10	3x12	3x12	3x15	3x15
	1b. REVERSE LUNGE *tempo:* 1-1-3 | *rest:* 30 sec	3x10	3x10	3x12	3x12	3x15	3x15
	2a. PLANK WALK-UP *tempo:* 1-1-2 | *rest:* 10 sec	3x8	3x8	3x10	3x10	3x10	3x10
	2b. STRAIGHT-LEG RAISE *tempo:* 1-1-3 | *rest:* 30 sec	3x8	3x8	3x10	3x10	3x12	3x12
	3a. DIP WITH BAR *tempo:* 1-1-2 | *rest:* 10 sec	3x8	3x8	3x10	3x10	3x12	3x12
	3b. SINGLE-LEG SQUAT *tempo:* 1-1-3 | *rest:* 30 sec	3x6	3x6	3x8	3x8	3x10	3x12
	4a. PUSH-UP *tempo:* 1-1-3 | *rest:* 10 sec	3x#	3x#+1	3x#+2	3x#+3	3x#+4	3x#+5
	4b. ALTERNATE SINGLE-LEG RAISE *tempo:* 1-1-2 | *rest:* 30 sec	3x8	3x8	3x10	3x10	3x12	3x12
	5a. FRAME-ASSISTED SIT-UP *tempo:* 1-1-3 | *rest:* 10 sec	3x10	3x10	3x10	3x12	3x12	3x12
	5b. REVERSE LUNGE *tempo:* 1-1-3 | *rest:* 30 sec	3x10	3x12	3x12	3x12	3x12	3x13

GENERAL FITNESS (INTERMEDIATE)

PREREQUISITE: General Fitness (Beginner) (page 51) or scoring average or better on push-ups (page 37) and pull-ups (page 37)

MACROCYCLE: *Three six-week mesocycles:* Single Set, Superset, Trisets. *Extras:* cardio 2–3 days/week.

	SINGLE SET	WEEK 1 set x rep	WEEK 2 set x rep	WEEK 3 set x rep	WEEK 4 set x rep	WEEK 5 set x rep	WEEK 6 set x rep
DAY 1	**STANDARD PULL-UP** tempo: 1-1-3 | rest: 60 sec	3x8	3x8	3x10	3x10	3x10	3x12
	PUSH-UP tempo: 1-1-3 | rest: 60 sec	3x10	3x10	3x12	3x15	3x20	3x20
	PRESS-UP tempo: 1-1-2 | rest: 60 sec	3x8	3x8	3x10	3x12	3x12	3x12
	WIDE-GRIP PULL-UP tempo: 1-1-3 | rest: 60 sec	3x6	3x6	3x7	3x8	3x8	3x9
	DIP WITH BAR tempo: 1-1-2 | rest: 45 sec	3x8	3x9	3x9	3x10	3x10	3x12
	WIDE PUSH-UP tempo: 1-1-3 | rest: 60 sec	3x10	3x10	3x12	3x12	3x15	3x15
	PIKE PRESS tempo: 1-1-3 | rest: 60 sec	3x6	3x6	3x8	3x8	3x10	3x10
	CLOSE-GRIP PULL-UP tempo: 1-1-3 | rest: 60 sec	3x5	3x5	3x6	3x7	3x7	3x8
DAY 2	**SQUAT** tempo: 1-1-3 | rest: 45 sec	3x15	3x15	3x20	3x20	3x25	3x25
	SPLIT SQUAT tempo: 1-1-3 | rest: 45 sec	3x10	3x10	3x12	3x12	3x15	3x15
	FORWARD LUNGE tempo: 1-1-3 | rest: 45 sec	3x8	3x10	3x12	3x12	3x15	3x15
	SINGLE-LEG SQUAT tempo: 1-1-3 | rest: 45 sec	3x8	3x10	3x10	3x10	3x12	3x12
	HANGING LEG RAISE tempo: 1-1-3 | rest: 60 sec	3x8	3x8	3x10	3x12	3x12	3x12
	HANGING BICYCLE tempo: 1-1-1 | rest: 60 sec	3x12	3x12	3x12	3x12	3x15	3x15
	HIGH TWIST tempo: 1-1-2 | rest: 60 sec	3x6	3x8	3x10	3x10	3x12	3x12
	LEG CURL WITH EXTENSION tempo: 1-1-3 | rest: 60 sec	3x8	3x8	3x10	3x10	3x10	3x12

DAY 3		WEEK 1	WEEK 2	WEEK 3	WEEK 4	WEEK 5	WEEK 6
	FLOOR DIP *tempo: 1-1-2 | rest: 45 sec*	3x10	3x10	3x12	3x12	3x15	3x15
	PARALLEL GRIP PULL-UP *tempo: 1-1-3 | rest: 60 sec*	3x8	3x8	3x8	3x10	3x10	3x10
	ALTERNATE-GRIP PULL-UP *tempo: 1-1-3 | rest: 60 sec*	3x6	3x6	3x6	3x6	3x6	3x7
	STAGGERED PUSH-UP *tempo: 1-1-3 | rest: 60 sec*	3x10	3x12	3x12	3x12	3x12	3x12
	BICYCLE CRUNCH *tempo: 1-1-3 | rest: 45 sec*	3x10	3x12	3x12	3x15	3x15	3x15
	HANGING LEG CURL *tempo: 1-1-3 | rest: 45 sec*	3x10	3x10	3x12	3x12	3x15	3x15
	HANGING OBLIQUE CRUNCH *tempo: 1-1-2 | rest: 45 sec*	3x6	3x8	3x8	3x10	3x10	3x12
	TOTAL-BODY CRUNCH *tempo: 1-1-2 | rest: 60 sec*	3x8	3x10	3x12	3x12	3x15	3x15

	SUPERSETS	WEEK 1 set x rep	WEEK 2 set x rep	WEEK 3 set x rep	WEEK 4 set x rep	WEEK 5 set x rep	WEEK 6 set x rep
DAY 1	**1a. POWER PUSH-UP** *tempo: 1-1-3 | rest: 10 sec*	3x8	3x8	3x10	3x10	3x10	3x12
	1b. SQUAT *tempo: 1-1-3 | rest: 30 sec*	3x12	3x12	3x15	3x15	3x15	3x20
	2a. SIDE-TO-SIDE PULL-UP *tempo: 1-1-3 | rest: 10 sec*	3x4	3x4	3x5	3x5	3x6	3x6
	2b. LEG EXTENSION *tempo: 1-1-3 | rest: 30 sec*	3x10	3x10	3x12	3x12	3x15	3x15
	3a. ALTERNATE-GRIP PUSH-UP W/BAR *tempo: 1-1-3 | rest: 10 sec*	3x6	3x6	3x6	3x7	3x7	3x7
	3b. CALF RAISE *tempo: 1-1-2 | rest: 30 sec*	3x8	3x8	3x10	3x10	3x12	3x12
	4a. STANDARD PULL-UP *tempo: 1-1-3 | rest: 10 sec*	3x10	3x10	3x10	3x10	3x12	3x10
	4b. SINGLE-LEG SQUAT *tempo: 1-1-2 | rest: 30 sec*	3x8	3x8	3x10	3x10	3x12	3x12
	5a. DIP WITH BAR *tempo: 1-1-2 | rest: 10 sec*	3x12	3x12	3x12	3x15	3x15	3x15
	5b. SINGLE-LEG BRIDGE *tempo: 1-1-2 | rest: 30 sec*	3x10	3x10	3x12	3x12	3x12	3x15

1a. SQUAT JUMP *tempo:* fast | *rest:* 10 sec	3x10	3x10	3x12	3x12	3x15	3x15
1b. HANGING LEG CURL W/ROTATION *tempo:* 1-1-3 | *rest:* 10 sec	3x8	3x10	3x10	3x12	3x12	3x15
2a. SKATER *tempo:* fast | *rest:* 10 sec	3x12	3x12	3x15	3x15	3x15	3x20
2b. PLANK TO SIDE PLANK *tempo:* 1-1-2 | *rest:* 10 sec	3x10	3x10	3x10	3x12	3x12	3x12
3a. REVERSE LUNGE *tempo:* 1-1-3 | *rest:* 10 sec	3x8	3x8	3x10	3x10	3x12	3x12
3b. HALF CIRCLE *tempo:* 1-1-3 | *rest:* 30 sec	3x10	3x10	3x12	3x12	3x12	3x12
4a. SINGLE-LEG SQUAT *tempo:* 1-1-3 | *rest:* 10 sec	3x10	3x10	3x12	3x12	3x12	3x15
4b. TOTAL-BODY CRUNCH *tempo:* 1-1-2 | *rest:* 10 sec	3x10	3x10	3x12	3x12	3x12	3x15
5a. SPLIT SQUAT *tempo:* 1-1-3 | *rest:* 10 sec	3x10	3x10	3x12	3x12	3x15	3x15
5b. PLANK *tempo:* 1-45-1 | *rest:* 10 sec	3x1	3x1	3x1	3x1	3x1	3x1
1a. PRESS-UP WITH PULL-UP BAR *tempo:* 1-1-2 | *rest:* 10 sec	3x8	3x10	3x10	3x12	3x12	3x15
1b. CORE WALK-OUT *tempo:* 1-1-3 | *rest:* 10 sec	3x10	3x10	3x10	3x10	3x12	3x15
2a. TRICEPS PUSH-UP *tempo:* 1-1-3 | *rest:* 10 sec	3x10	3x12	3x12	3x15	3x15	3x15
2b. OBLIQUE TWIST *tempo:* 1-1-2 | *rest:* 10 sec	3x8	3x8	3x10	3x10	3x12	3x12
3a. CHIN-UP *tempo:* 1-1-3 | *rest:* 10 sec	3x10	3x10	3x11	3x12	3x12	3x12
3b. HANGING OBLIQUE CRUNCH *tempo:* 1-1-3 | *rest:* 30 sec	3x6	3x7	3x7	3x8	3x8	3x8
4a. FLOOR DIP *tempo:* 1-1-2 | *rest:* 10 sec	3x12	3x12	3x12	3x15	3x15	3x15
4b. LEG CURL *tempo:* 1-1-3 | *rest:* 10 sec	3x12	3x12	3x12	3x12	3x15	3x15
5a. STAGGERED PUSH-UP *tempo:* 1-1-3 | *rest:* 10 sec	3x10	3x10	3x11	3x11	3x12	3x12
5b. CRUNCH *tempo:* 1-1-2 | *rest:* 30 sec	3x25	3x25	3x30	3x30	3x30	3x30

DAY 2 (rows 1a–5b PLANK)

DAY 3 (rows 1a PRESS-UP–5b CRUNCH)

TRISETS		WEEK 1 set x rep	WEEK 2 set x rep	WEEK 3 set x rep	WEEK 4 set x rep	WEEK 5 set x rep	WEEK 6 set x rep
DAY 1	**1a. CHIN-UP** *tempo:* 1-1-3 | *rest:* 10 sec	3x10	3x10	3x10	3x11	3x11	3x12
	1b. SQUAT *tempo:* 1-1-3 | *rest:* 10 sec	3x20	3x20	3x20	3x20	3x20	3x20
	1c. TOTAL-BODY CRUNCH *tempo:* 1-1-2 | *rest:* 30 sec	3x12	3x12	3x12	3x15	3x15	3x15
	2a. PULL-UP WITH LEG CURL *tempo:* 1-1-3 | *rest:* 10 sec	3x6	3x6	3x8	3x8	3x8	3x8
	2b. SPLIT SQUAT *tempo:* 1-1-3 | *rest:* 10 sec	3x8	3x8	3x8	3x10	3x10	3x10
	2c. PLANK *tempo:* 1-60-3 | *rest:* 30 sec	3x1	3x1	3x1	3x1	3x1	3x1
	3a. POWER PUSH-UP *tempo:* fast | *rest:* 10 sec	3x8	3x10	3x10	3x12	3x12	3x12
	3b. SINGLE-LEG BRIDGE *tempo:* 1-1-3 | *rest:* 30 sec	3x8	3x8	3x10	3x10	3x12	3x12
	3c. FRAME-ASSISTED SIT-UP *tempo:* 1-1-3 | *rest:* 30 sec	3x10	3x10	3x10	3x12	3x12	3x12
	4a. PRESS-UP *tempo:* 1-1-2 | *rest:* 10 sec	3x10	3x10	3x12	3x12	3x15	3x15
	4b. CALF RAISE *tempo:* 1-1-2 | *rest:* 10 sec	3x15	3x15	3x15	3x15	3x15	3x15
	4c. REVERSE LUNGE *tempo:* 1-1-3 | *rest:* 30 sec	3x10	3x10	3x10	3x10	3x10	3x10
DAY 2	**1a. DIP WITH BAR** *tempo:* 1-1-2 | *rest:* 10 sec	3x10	3x12	3x12	3x12	3x15	3x15
	1b. FORWARD LUNGE *tempo:* 1-1-3 | *rest:* 10 sec	3x12	3x12	3x12	3x12	3x12	3x12
	1c. STRAIGHT-LEG RAISE SIDE TO SIDE *tempo:* 1-1-3 | *rest:* 30 sec	3x8	3x8	3x8	3x10	3x10	3x10
	2a. STANDING WALK-OUT *tempo:* 1-1-3 | *rest:* 10 sec	3x10	3x10	3x10	3x10	3x10	3x10
	2b. SKATER *tempo:* fast | *rest:* 10 sec	3x20	3x20	3x20	3x20	3x20	3x20
	2C. HANGING LEG CURL *tempo:* 1-1-3 | *rest:* 30 sec	3x8	3x10	3x10	3x12	3x12	3x12
	3a. SIDE-TO-SIDE PULL-UP *tempo:* 1-1-3 | *rest:* 10 sec	3x4	3x4	3x5	3x5	3x6	3x6
	3b. LEG EXTENSION *tempo:* 1-1-3 | *rest:* 30 sec	3x15	3x15	3x15	3x15	3x15	3x15
	3c. PLANK *tempo:* 1-60-1 | *rest:* 30 sec	3x1	3x1	3x1	3x1	3x1	3x1
	4a. SHORT-RANGE PULL-UP (UPPER) *tempo:* 1-1-3 | *rest:* 10 sec	3x10	3x10	3x10	3x12	3x12	3x12
	4b. SINGLE-LEG SQUAT *tempo:* 1-1-3 | *rest:* 10 sec	3x8	3x8	3x10	3x10	3x12	3x12
	4c. SIDE PLANK *tempo:* 1-1-3 | *rest:* 30 sec	3x8	3x8	3x10	3x10	3x12	3x12

1a. PRESS-UP WITH PULL-UP BAR *tempo:* 1-1-2 | *rest:* 10 sec	3x10	3x10	3x102	3x12	3x12	3x12
1b. SQUAT JUMP *tempo:* fast | *rest:* 10 sec	3x10	3x12	3x12	3x15	3x15	3x15
1c. LEG CURL WITH EXTENSION *tempo:* 1-1-2 | *rest:* 30 sec	3x8	3x8	3x10	3x12	3x12	3x12
2a. ALTERNATE-GRIP PUSH-UP W/BAR *tempo:* 1-1-3 | *rest:* 10 sec	3x6	3x6	3x8	3x8	3x80	3x10
2b. SPLIT SQUAT *tempo:* 1-1-3 | *rest:* 10 sec	3x8	3x8	3x8	3x10	3x10	3x12
2C. FULL CIRCLE *tempo:* 1-1-2 | *rest:* 30 sec	3x5	3x6	3x6	3x6	3x7	3x7
3a. DIAMOND PUSH-UP *tempo:* 1-1-3 | *rest:* 10 sec	3x10	3x10	3x10	3x12	3x12	3x12
3b. REVERSE LUNGE *tempo:* 1-1-3 | *rest:* 10 sec	3x12	3x12	3x12	3x12	3x12	3x12
3c. BICYCLE CRUNCH *tempo:* 1-1-1 | *rest:* 30 sec	3x12	3x12	3x15	3x15	3x15	3x15
4a. ALTERNATE-GRIP PULL-UP *tempo:* 1-1-3 | *rest:* 10 sec	3x5	3x5	3x6	3x6	3x7	3x7
4b. FORWARD LUNGE *tempo:* 1-1-3 | *rest:* 10 sec	3x8	3x10	3x10	3x120	3x12	3x12
4c. TOTAL-BODY CRUNCH *tempo:* 1-1-2 | *rest:* 30 sec	3x10	3x10	3x12	3x12	3x12	3x12

(DAY 3)

WEIGHT LOSS (BEGINNER)

PREREQUISITE: There are no prerequisites for the beginner program.

MACROCYCLE: *Three six-week mesocycles:* Single Set, Trisets, Timed Circuit. *Extras:* cardio 3–4 days/week for 30–40 min moderate intensity.

SINGLE SET		WEEK 1 set x rep	WEEK 2 set x rep	WEEK 3 set x rep	WEEK 4 set x rep	WEEK 5 set x rep	WEEK 6 set x rep
DAY 1	**CHIN-UP** tempo: 1-1-3 | rest: 60 sec	2x5	2x5	3x5	3x5	3x6	3x6
	PUSH-UP tempo: 1-1-3 | rest: 60 sec	2x#	2x#+1	3x#+2	3x#+3	3x#+4	3x#+4
	DIP WITH BAR tempo: 1-1-2 | rest: 60 sec	2x8	2x8	3x8	3x8	3x10	3x10
	STANDARD PULL-UP tempo: 1-1-3 | rest: 60 sec	2x#	2x#+1	3x#+1	3x#+2	3x#+2	3x#+2
	PLANK WALK-UP tempo: 1-1-1 | rest: 30 sec	2x5	2x5	3x5	3x6	3x6	3x7
	DIAMOND PUSH-UP tempo: 1-1-2 | rest: 45 sec	2x8	2x8	3x8	3x10	3x10	3x10
	STANDING WALK-OUT tempo: 1-1-3 | rest: 45 sec	2x8	2x8	3x10	3x10	3x12	3x12
	PARALLEL GRIP PULL-UP tempo: 1-1-3 | rest: 60 sec	2x4	2x4	3x4	3x5	3x5	3x6
DAY 2	**SQUAT** tempo: 1-1-3 | rest: 45 sec	2x10	2x12	3x15	3x15	3x15	3x20
	FORWARD LUNGE tempo: 1-1-2 | rest: 45 sec	2x8	2x8	3x10	3x10	3x12	3x12
	CALF RAISE tempo: 1-1-2 | rest: 45 sec	2x12	2x12	3x12	3x15	3x15	3x15
	BRIDGE tempo: 1-1-2 | rest: 30 sec	2x8	2x8	3x8	3x10	3x10	3x12
	CORE WALK-OUT tempo: 1-1-3 | rest: 30 sec	2x10	2x10	3x10	3x12	3x12	3x15
	PLANK tempo: 1-30-1 | rest: 30 sec	2x1	2x1	3x1	3x1	3x1	3x1
	SIDE PLANK tempo: 1-15-1 | rest: 30 sec	2x1	2x1	3x1	3x1	3x1	3x1
	STRAIGHT-LEG RAISE tempo: 1-1-3 | rest: 30 sec	2x8	2x8	3x8	3x8	3x8	3x8
DAY 3	**SIDE-FACING PULL-UP** tempo: 1-1-3 | rest: 60 sec	2x4	2x4	3x4	3x5	3x5	3x6
	CHAIR DIP tempo: 1-1-2 | rest: 45 sec	2x8	2x10	3x10	3x10	3x12	3x12
	ALTERNATE-GRIP PULL-UP tempo: 1-1-3 | rest: 60 sec	2x3	2x3	3x4	3x4	3x5	3x5
	PUSH-UP tempo: 1-1-3 | rest: 45 sec	2x5	2x6	3x6	3x7	3x8	3x8
	CRUNCH tempo: 1-1-2 | rest: 30 sec	2x20	2x20	3x20	3x20	3x20	3x20
	LEG CURL tempo: 1-1-2 | rest: 30 sec	2x10	2x10	3x10	3x12	3x12	3x12
	BICYCLE CRUNCH tempo: 1-1-1 | rest: 30 sec	2x10	2x12	3x12	3x12	3x12	3x15
	HANGING LEG CURL tempo: 1-1-3 | rest: 30 sec	2x8	2x8	3x8	3x10	3x10	3x12

TRISETS	WEEK 1 *set x rep*	WEEK 2 *set x rep*	WEEK 3 *set x rep*	WEEK 4 *set x rep*	WEEK 5 *set x rep*	WEEK 6 *set x rep*
1a. HIGH KNEES *tempo:* fast | *rest:* 30 sec	2x30 sec	2x30 sec	3x30 sec	3x30 sec	3x30 sec	3x30 sec
1b. CHIN-UP *tempo:* 1-1-3 | *rest:* 20 sec	2x6	2x6	3x6	3x7	3x7	3x7
1c. CRUNCH *tempo:* 1-1-2 | *rest:* 20 sec	2x20	2x20	3x20	3x25	3x25	3x25
2a. SKATER *tempo:* fast | *rest:* 30 sec	2x30 sec	2x30 sec	3x30 sec	3x30 sec	3x30 sec	3x30 sec
2b. PUSH-UP *tempo:* 1-1-3 | *rest:* 20 sec	2x#	2x#	3x#	3x#+1	3x#+2	3x#+3
2c. HANGING LEG CURL *tempo:* 1-1-3 | *rest:* 20 sec	2x10	2x10	3x10	3x12	3x12	3x12
3a. SPEED SQUAT *tempo:* fast | *rest:* 30 sec	2x20	2x20	3x20	3x20	3x20	3x20
3b. DIP *tempo:* 1-1-2 | *rest:* 20 sec	2x10	2x10	3x10	3x10	3x12	3x12
3c. CORE WALK-OUT *tempo:* 1-1-3 | *rest:* 20 sec	2x10	2x10	3x10	3x12	3x12	3x12
4a. MOUNTAIN CLIMBER *tempo:* fast | *rest:* 30 sec	2x30 sec	2x30 sec	3x30 sec	3x30 sec	3x30 sec	3x30 sec
4b. STAGGERED PUSH-UP *tempo:* 1-1-3 | *rest:* 20 sec	2x8	2x8	3x8	3x10	3x10	3x12
4c. FRAME-ASSISTED SIT-UP *tempo:* 1-1-3 | *rest:* 20 sec	2x10	2x10	3x10	3x12	3x12	3x12
1a. SQUAT JUMP *tempo:* fast | *rest:* 30 sec	2x10	2x10	3x10	3x10	3x10	3x10
1b. STANDARD PULL-UP *tempo:* 1-1-3 | *rest:* 20 sec	2x#	2x#	3x#	3x#+1	3x#+1	3x#+2
1c. HANGING LEG RAISE *tempo:* 1-1-3 | *rest:* 20 sec	2x10	2x10	3x10	3x12	3x12	3x12
2a. SHOULDER TOUCH *tempo:* fast | *rest:* 30 sec	2x12	2x12	3x12	3x12	3x12	3x12
2b. DIAMOND PUSH-UP *tempo:* 1-1-3 | *rest:* 20 sec	2x12	2x12	3x12	3x12	3x15	3x15
2c. HANGING OBLIQUE CRUNCH *tempo:* 1-1-2 | *rest:* 20 sec	2x8	2x8	3x8	3x8	3x10	3x10
3a. JUMPING LUNGE *tempo:* fast | *rest:* 30 sec	2x8	2x8	3x8	3x8	3x8	3x8
3b. CHAIR DIP *tempo:* 1-1-2 | *rest:* 20 sec	2x10	2x10	3x10	3x12	3x12	3x12
3c. TOTAL-BODY CRUNCH *tempo:* 1-1-2 | *rest:* 20 sec	2x10	2x10	3x10	3x12	3x12	3x12
4a. HIGH KNEES *tempo:* fast | *rest:* 30 sec	2x30 sec	2x30 sec	3x30 sec	3x30 sec	3x30 sec	3x30 sec
4b. SHORT-RANGE PULL-UP (UPPER) *tempo:* 1-1-3 | *rest:* 20 sec	2x5	2x5	3x5	3x6	3x6	3x6
4c. PLANK *tempo:* 1-45-1 | *rest:* 20 sec	2x1	2x1	3x1	3x1	3x1	3x1

DAY 1 (rows 1a–4c FRAME-ASSISTED SIT-UP)
DAY 2 (rows 1a SQUAT JUMP–4c PLANK)

DAY 3							
1a. SPEED SQUAT *tempo:* fast | *rest:* 30 sec	2x20	2x20	3x20	3x20	3x20	3x20
1b. PARALLEL GRIP PULL-UP *tempo:* 1-1-3 | *rest:* 20 sec	2x5	2x5	3x5	3x6	3x6	3x7
1c. SPLIT SQUAT *tempo:* 1-1-3 | *rest:* 20 sec	2x8	2x8	3x8	3x8	3x10	3x10
2a. MOUNTAIN CLIMBER *tempo:* fast | *rest:* 30 sec	2x30 sec	2x30 sec	3x30 sec	3x30 sec	3x30 sec	3x30 sec
2b. PUSH-UP *tempo:* 1-1-3 | *rest:* 20 sec	2x8	2x8	3x8	3x10	3x10	3x10
2C. SINGLE-LEG BRIDGE *tempo:* 1-1-2 | *rest:* 20 sec	2x8	2x8	3x8	3x10	3x12	3x12
3a. JUMPING LUNGE *tempo:* fast | *rest:* 30 sec	2x8	2x8	3x8	3x10	3x10	3x10
3b. PLANK WALK-UP *tempo:* 1-1-2 | *rest:* 20 sec	2x6	2x6	3x6	3x7	3x7	3x8
3c. CALF RAISE *tempo:* 1-1-2 | *rest:* 20 sec	2x12	2x12	3x12	3x15	3x15	3x15
4a. SKATER *tempo:* fast | *rest:* 30 sec	2x30 sec	2x30 sec	3x30 sec	3x30 sec	3x30 sec	3x30 sec
4b. FLOOR DIP *tempo:* 1-1-2 | *rest:* 20 sec	2x10	2x10	3x10	3x10	3x12	3x12
4c. REVERSE LUNGE *tempo:* 1-1-3 | *rest:* 20 sec	2x8	2x8	3x8	3x10	3x10	3x12

	TIMED CIRCUIT	**WEEK 1** duration	**WEEK 2** duration	**WEEK 3** duration	**WEEK 4** duration	**WEEK 5** duration	**WEEK 6** duration
DAY 1	**HIGH KNEES** *rest:* 30 sec	30 sec	30 sec	35 sec	35 sec	40 sec	40 sec
	CHIN-UP *rest:* 30 sec	30 sec	30 sec	35 sec	35 sec	40 sec	40 sec
	SQUAT *rest:* 30 sec	30 sec	30 sec	35 sec	35 sec	40 sec	40 sec
	BICYCLE CRUNCH *rest:* 30 sec	30 sec	30 sec	35 sec	35 sec	40 sec	40 sec
	SKATER *rest:* 30 sec	30 sec	30 sec	35 sec	35 sec	40 sec	40 sec
	PUSH-UP *rest:* 30 sec	30 sec	30 sec	35 sec	35 sec	40 sec	40 sec
	FORWARD LUNGE *rest:* 30 sec	30 sec	30 sec	35 sec	35 sec	40 sec	40 sec
	HANGING LEG RAISE *rest:* 30 sec	30 sec	30 sec	35 sec	35 sec	40 sec	40 sec
	ROUNDS	2	3	2	3	2	3

DAY 2	**MOUNTAIN CLIMBER** *rest:* 30 sec	30 sec	30 sec	35 sec	35 sec	40 sec	40 sec
	PARALLEL GRIP PULL-UP *rest:* 30 sec	30 sec	30 sec	35 sec	35 sec	40 sec	40 sec
	SINGLE-LEG BRIDGE *rest:* 30 sec	30 sec	30 sec	35 sec	35 sec	40 sec	40 sec
	PLANK *rest:* 30 sec	30 sec	30 sec	35 sec	35 sec	40 sec	40 sec
	SPEED SQUAT *rest:* 30 sec	30 sec	30 sec	35 sec	35 sec	40 sec	40 sec
	DIP WITH BAR *rest:* 30 sec	30 sec	30 sec	35 sec	35 sec	40 sec	40 sec
	LEG EXTENSION *rest:* 30 sec	30 sec	30 sec	35 sec	35 sec	40 sec	40 sec
	FRAME-ASSISTED SIT-UP *rest:* 30 sec	30 sec	30 sec	35 sec	35 sec	40 sec	40 sec
	ROUNDS	2	3	2	3	2	3
DAY 3	**SINGLE-LEG SQUAT** *rest:* 30 sec	30 sec	30 sec	35 sec	35 sec	40 sec	40 sec
	HANGING OBLIQUE CRUNCH *rest:* 30 sec	30 sec	30 sec	35 sec	35 sec	40 sec	40 sec
	JUMPING LUNGE *rest:* 30 sec	30 sec	30 sec	35 sec	35 sec	40 sec	40 sec
	PRESS-UP *rest:* 30 sec	30 sec	30 sec	35 sec	35 sec	40 sec	40 sec
	REVERSE LUNGE *rest:* 30 sec	30 sec	30 sec	35 sec	35 sec	40 sec	40 sec
	STRAIGHT-LEG RAISE *rest:* 30 sec	30 sec	30 sec	35 sec	35 sec	40 sec	40 sec
	ROUNDS	2	3	2	3	2	3

WEIGHT LOSS (INTERMEDIATE)

PREREQUISITE: Weight Loss (Beginner) (page 58) or average 1.5-mile run time (page 39) and average chair squat (page 38)

MACROCYCLE: *Three six-week mesocycles:* Trisets, Timed Circuit 1, Timed Circuit 2. *Extras:* cardio 3–4 days/week for 30 min moderate to high intensity.

	TRISETS	WEEK 1 set x rep	WEEK 2 set x rep	WEEK 3 set x rep	WEEK 4 set x rep	WEEK 5 set x rep	WEEK 6 set x rep
	1a. HIGH KNEES *tempo:* fast | *rest:* 20 sec	3x30 sec	3x30 sec	3x35 sec	3x35 sec	3x40 sec	3x40 sec
	1b. CHIN-UP *tempo:* 1-1-3 | *rest:* 10 sec	3x8	3x8	3x9	3x9	3x10	3x10
	1c. STRAIGHT-LEG RAISE SIDE TO SIDE *tempo:* 1-1-2 | *rest:* 30 sec	3x5	3x5	3x6	3x6	3x7	3x7
	2a. SKATER *tempo:* fast | *rest:* 20 sec	3x30 sec	3x30 sec	3x35 sec	3x35 sec	3x40 sec	3x40 sec
	2b. PUSH-UP *tempo:* 1-1-3 | *rest:* 10 sec	3x10	3x12	3x15	3x15	3x20	3x20
	2c. HANGING LEG CURL *tempo:* 1-1-2 | *rest:* 10 sec	3x10	3x12	3x12	3x12	3x15	3x15
DAY 1	**3a. SPEED SQUAT** *tempo:* fast | *rest:* 20 sec	3x30 sec	3x30 sec	3x35 sec	3x35 sec	3x40 sec	3x40 sec
	3b. PIKE PRESS *tempo:* 1-1-3 | *rest:* 10 sec	3x8	3x8	3x10	3x10	3x12	3x12
	3c. CORE WALK-OUT *tempo:* 1-1-3 | *rest:* 10 sec	3x8	3x8	3x10	3x10	3x10	3x10
	4a. MOUNTAIN CLIMBER *tempo:* fast | *rest:* 20 sec	3x30 sec	3x30 sec	3x35 sec	3x35 sec	3x40 sec	3x40 sec
	4b. STAGGERED PUSH-UP *tempo:* 1-1-3 | *rest:* 10 sec	3x6	3x6	3x8	3x8	3x10	3x10
	4c. FRAME-ASSISTED SIT-UP *tempo:* 1-1-3 | *rest:* 10 sec	3x10	3x10	3x12	3x12	3x12	3x15

	Exercise						
DAY 2	**1a. SQUAT JUMP** *tempo:* fast | *rest:* 20 sec	3x10	3x10	3x15	3x15	3x20	3x20
	1b. STANDARD PULL-UP *tempo:* 1-1-3 | *rest:* 10 sec	3x8	3x10	3x10	3x12	3x12	3x15
	1c. LEG CURL WITH EXTENSION *tempo:* 1-1-3 | *rest:* 30 sec	3x8	3x10	3x10	3x12	3x12	3x12
	2a. SHOULDER TOUCH *tempo:* fast | *rest:* 20 sec	3x10	3x10	3x15	3x15	3x15	3x15
	2b. POWER PUSH-UP *tempo:* fast | *rest:* 10 sec	3x8	3x8	3x10	3x12	3x12	3x12
	2C. HANGING OBLIQUE CRUNCH *tempo:* 1-1-2 | *rest:* 10 sec	3x8	3x8	3x10	3x10	3x10	3x10
	3a. JUMPING LUNGE *tempo:* fast | *rest:* 20 sec	3x10	3x10	3x10	3x12	3x15	3x15
	3b. CHAIR DIP *tempo:* 1-1-3 | *rest:* 10 sec	3x12	3x12	3x12	3x15	3x15	3x15
	3c. TOTAL-BODY CRUNCH *tempo:* 1-1-2 | *rest:* 10 sec	3x12	3x12	3x12	3x12	3x15	3x15
	4a. HIGH KNEES *tempo:* fast | *rest:* 20 sec	3x30 sec	3x30 sec	3x35 sec	3x35 sec	3x40 sec	3x40 sec
	4b. SHORT-RANGE PULL-UP (UPPER) *tempo:* 1-1-2 | *rest:* 10 sec	3x8	3x10	3x12	3x12	3x15	3x15
	4c. HALF CIRCLE *tempo:* 1-1-2 | *rest:* 10 sec	3x6	3x6	3x7	3x8	3x8	3x8
DAY 3	**1a. SQUAT THRUST** *tempo:* fast | *rest:* 20 sec	3x10	3x10	3x12	3x15	3x20	3x20
	1b. PARALLEL GRIP PULL-UP *tempo:* 1-1-3 | *rest:* 10 sec	3x8	3x10	3x10	3x12	3x12	3x12
	1c. SPLIT SQUAT *tempo:* 1-1-3 | *rest:* 10 sec	3x8	3x8	3x9	3x10	3x10	3x12
	2a. MOUNTAIN CLIMBER *tempo:* fast | *rest:* 20 sec	3x30 sec	3x30 sec	3x35 sec	3x35 sec	3x40 sec	3x40 sec
	2b. PUSH-UP *tempo:* 1-1-3 | *rest:* 10 sec	3x12	3x12	3x15	3x15	3x20	3x20
	2C. SINGLE-LEG BRIDGE *tempo:* 1-1-2 | *rest:* 10 sec	3x10	3x10	3x10	3x12	3x12	3x15
	3a. JUMPING LUNGE *tempo:* fast | *rest:* 20 sec	3x10	3x10	3x10	3x12	3x15	3x15
	3b. PLANK WALK-UP *tempo:* 1-1-3 | *rest:* 10 sec	3x6	3x7	3x8	3x9	3x10	3x12
	3c. CALF RAISE *tempo:* 1-1-2 | *rest:* 10 sec	3x10	3x10	3x12	3x15	3x15	3x15
	4a. SKATER *tempo:* fast | *rest:* 10 sec	3x30 sec	3x30 sec	3x35 sec	3x35 sec	3x40 sec	3x40 sec
	4b. STANDING WALK-OUT *tempo:* 1-1-3 | *rest:* 10 sec	3x10	3x12	3x12	3x12	3x12	3x15
	4c. REVERSE LUNGE *tempo:* 1-1-3 | *rest:* 10 sec	3x8	3x10	3x10	3x12	3x12	3x15

TIMED CIRCUIT 1		WEEK 1 duration	WEEK 2 duration	WEEK 3 duration	WEEK 4 duration	WEEK 5 duration	WEEK 6 duration
DAY 1	**HIGH KNEES** *rest: 25 sec*	35 sec	35 sec	40 sec	40 sec	45 sec	45 sec
	CHIN-UP *rest: 25 sec*	35 sec	35 sec	40 sec	40 sec	45 sec	45 sec
	SQUAT *rest: 25 sec*	35 sec	35 sec	40 sec	40 sec	45 sec	45 sec
	BICYCLE CRUNCH *rest: 25 sec*	35 sec	35 sec	40 sec	40 sec	45 sec	45 sec
	SKATER *rest: 25 sec*	35 sec	35 sec	40 sec	40 sec	45 sec	45 sec
	PUSH-UP *rest: 25 sec*	35 sec	35 sec	40 sec	40 sec	45 sec	45 sec
	FORWARD LUNGE *rest: 25 sec*	35 sec	35 sec	40 sec	40 sec	45 sec	45 sec
	ALTERNATE SINGLE-LEG RAISE *rest: 25 sec*	35 sec	35 sec	40 sec	40 sec	45 sec	45 sec
	ROUNDS	3	3	3	3	3	3
DAY 2	**MOUNTAIN CLIMBER** *rest: 25 sec*	35 sec	35 sec	40 sec	40 sec	45 sec	45 sec
	PARALLEL GRIP PULL-UP *rest: 25 sec*	35 sec	35 sec	40 sec	40 sec	45 sec	45 sec
	SINGLE-LEG BRIDGE *rest: 25 sec*	35 sec	35 sec	40 sec	40 sec	45 sec	45 sec
	PLANK *rest: 25 sec*	35 sec	35 sec	40 sec	40 sec	45 sec	45 sec
	SPEED SQUAT *rest: 25 sec*	35 sec	35 sec	40 sec	40 sec	45 sec	45 sec
	PIKE PRESS *rest: 25 sec*	35 sec	35 sec	40 sec	40 sec	45 sec	45 sec
	LEG EXTENSION *rest: 25 sec*	35 sec	35 sec	40 sec	40 sec	45 sec	45 sec
	FRAME-ASSISTED SIT-UP *rest: 25 sec*	35 sec	35 sec	40 sec	40 sec	45 sec	45 sec
	ROUNDS	3	3	3	3	3	3

DAY 3		WEEK 1	WEEK 2	WEEK 3	WEEK 4	WEEK 5	WEEK 6
	SQUAT THRUST *rest:* 25 sec	35 sec	35 sec	40 sec	40 sec	45 sec	45 sec
	STANDARD PULL-UP *rest:* 25 sec	35 sec	35 sec	40 sec	40 sec	45 sec	45 sec
	SINGLE-LEG SQUAT *rest:* 25 sec	35 sec	35 sec	40 sec	40 sec	45 sec	45 sec
	HANGING OBLIQUE CRUNCH *rest:* 25 sec	35 sec	35 sec	40 sec	40 sec	45 sec	45 sec
	JUMPING LUNGE *rest:* 25 sec	35 sec	35 sec	40 sec	40 sec	45 sec	45 sec
	PRESS-UP WITH PULL-UP BAR *rest:* 25 sec	35 sec	35 sec	40 sec	40 sec	45 sec	45 sec
	FORWARD LUNGE *rest:* 25 sec	35 sec	35 sec	40 sec	40 sec	45 sec	45 sec
	STRAIGHT-LEG RAISE *rest:* 25 sec	35 sec	35 sec	40 sec	40 sec	45 sec	45 sec
	ROUNDS	3	3	3	3	3	3

TIMED CIRCUIT 2		WEEK 1 duration	WEEK 2 duration	WEEK 3 duration	WEEK 4 duration	WEEK 5 duration	WEEK 6 duration
DAY 1	**SQUAT THRUST** *rest:* 20 sec	40 sec	40 sec	45 sec	45 sec	50 sec	50 sec
	STANDARD PULL-UP *rest:* 20 sec	40 sec	40 sec	45 sec	45 sec	50 sec	50 sec
	REVERSE LUNGE *rest:* 20 sec	40 sec	40 sec	45 sec	45 sec	50 sec	50 sec
	CHAIR DIP *rest:* 20 sec	40 sec	40 sec	45 sec	45 sec	50 sec	50 sec
	SPEED SQUAT *rest:* 20 sec	40 sec	40 sec	45 sec	45 sec	50 sec	50 sec
	HANGING LEG RAISE *rest:* 20 sec	40 sec	40 sec	45 sec	45 sec	50 sec	50 sec
	POWER PUSH-UP *rest:* 20 sec	40 sec	40 sec	45 sec	45 sec	50 sec	50 sec
	TOTAL-BODY CRUNCH *rest:* 30 sec	40 sec	40 sec	45 sec	45 sec	50 sec	50 sec
	SINGLE-LEG BRIDGE *rest:* 20 sec	40 sec	40 sec	45 sec	45 sec	50 sec	50 sec
	HIGH KNEES *rest:* 20 sec	40 sec	40 sec	45 sec	45 sec	50 sec	50 sec
	ROUNDS	3	3	3	3	3	3

DAY 2	**SQUAT JUMP** *rest: 20 sec*	40 sec	40 sec	45 sec	45 sec	50 sec	50 sec
	SIDE-FACING PULL-UP *rest: 20 sec*	40 sec	40 sec	45 sec	45 sec	50 sec	50 sec
	HANGING OBLIQUE CRUNCH *rest: 20 sec*	40 sec	40 sec	45 sec	45 sec	50 sec	50 sec
	SQUAT *rest: 20 sec*	40 sec	40 sec	45 sec	45 sec	50 sec	50 sec
	BICYCLE CRUNCH *rest: 20 sec*	40 sec	40 sec	45 sec	45 sec	50 sec	50 sec
	SKATER *rest: 20 sec*	40 sec	40 sec	45 sec	45 sec	50 sec	50 sec
	PLANK *rest: 20 sec*	40 sec	40 sec	45 sec	45 sec	50 sec	50 sec
	ALTERNATE-GRIP PUSH-UP WITH BAR *rest: 20 sec*	40 sec	40 sec	45 sec	45 sec	50 sec	50 sec
	DIP WITH BAR *rest: 20 sec*	40 sec	40 sec	45 sec	45 sec	50 sec	50 sec
	HIGH KNEES *rest: 20 sec*	40 sec	40 sec	45 sec	45 sec	50 sec	50 sec
	ROUNDS	3	3	3	3	3	3
DAY 3	**MOUNTAIN CLIMBER** *rest: 20 sec*	40 sec	40 sec	45 sec	45 sec	50 sec	50 sec
	SPLIT SQUAT *rest: 20 sec*	40 sec	40 sec	45 sec	45 sec	50 sec	50 sec
	STAGGERED PUSH-UP *rest: 20 sec*	40 sec	40 sec	45 sec	45 sec	50 sec	50 sec
	STRAIGHT-LEG RAISE *rest: 20 sec*	40 sec	40 sec	45 sec	45 sec	50 sec	50 sec
	SHOULDER TOUCH *rest: 20 sec*	40 sec	40 sec	45 sec	45 sec	50 sec	50 sec
	PARALLEL GRIP PULL-UP *rest: 20 sec*	40 sec	40 sec	45 sec	45 sec	50 sec	50 sec
	FRAME-ASSISTED SIT-UP *rest: 20 sec*	40 sec	40 sec	45 sec	45 sec	50 sec	50 sec
	PIKE PRESS *rest: 20 sec*	40 sec	40 sec	45 sec	45 sec	50 sec	50 sec
	SINGLE-LEG SQUAT *rest: 20 sec*	40 sec	40 sec	45 sec	45 sec	50 sec	50 sec
	JUMPING LUNGE *rest: 20 sec*	40 sec	40 sec	45 sec	45 sec	50 sec	50 sec
	ROUNDS	3	3	3	3	3	3

MUSCULAR STRENGTH (INTERMEDIATE)

PREREQUISITE: General Fitness (Intermediate) (page 54) or average push-ups (page 37) and pull-ups (page 37)

MACROCYCLE: *Three six-week mesocycles:* Single Set, Single Set (Slow Negative), Supersets (Compound). *Extras:* cardio 1–2 days/week. *Note:* Pay attention to the tempo of the individual exercises.

	SINGLE SET	WEEK 1 set x rep	WEEK 2 set x rep	WEEK 3 set x rep	WEEK 4 set x rep	WEEK 5 set x rep	WEEK 6 set x rep
DAY 1	**STANDARD PULL-UP** *tempo:* 1-1-3 | *rest:* 60 sec	3x10	3x10	3x10	3x12	3x12	3x12
	CHIN-UP *tempo:* 1-1-3 | *rest:* 60 sec	3x12	3x12	3x12	3x12	3x15	3x15
	PIKE PRESS *tempo:* 1-1-2 | *rest:* 60 sec	3x10	3x10	3x12	3x12	3x12	3x15
	PARALLEL GRIP PULL-UP *tempo:* 1-1-3 | *rest:* 60 sec	3x12	3x12	3x12	3x12	3x12	3x12
	WIDE PUSH-UP *tempo:* 1-1-3 | *rest:* 60 sec	3x12	3x15	3x15	3x15	3x15	3x15
	SQUAT *tempo:* 1-1-3 | *rest:* 60 sec	3x12	3x15	3x15	3x15	3x15	3x20
	SINGLE-LEG BRIDGE *tempo:* 1-1-3 | *rest:* 60 sec	3x8	3x10	3x10	3x12	3x12	3x12
	SPLIT SQUAT *tempo:* 1-1-3 | *rest:* 60 sec	3x10	3x10	3x12	3x12	3x12	3x15
	LEG EXTENSION *tempo:* 1-1-3 | *rest:* 60 sec	3x12	3x15	3x15	3x15	3x15	3x20

DAY 2		WEEK 1	WEEK 2	WEEK 3	WEEK 4	WEEK 5	WEEK 6
	HANGING BICEPS CURL *tempo:* 1-1-3 | *rest:* 60 sec	3x12	3x12	3x12	3x12	3x15	3x15
	DIP WITH BAR *tempo:* 1-1-3 | *rest:* 60 sec	3x12	3x12	3x12	3x12	3x12	3x12
	DIAMOND PUSH-UP *tempo:* 1-1-3 | *rest:* 60 sec	3x12	3x12	3x12	3x12	3x15	3x15
	SHORT-RANGE PULL-UP (LOWER) *tempo:* 1-1-3 | *rest:* 60 sec	3x12	3x12	3x12	3x12	3x12	3x12
	PRESS-UP *tempo:* 1-1-3 | *rest:* 60 sec	3x12	3x12	3x15	3x15	3x15	3x15
	FRAME-ASSISTED SIT-UP *tempo:* 1-1-1 | *rest:* 60 sec	3x12	3x12	3x12	3x12	3x15	3x15
	STRAIGHT-LEG RAISE *tempo:* 1-1-2 | *rest:* 60 sec	3x10	3x10	3x12	3x12	3x12	3x15
	SIDE PLANK *tempo:* 1-1-3 | *rest:* 60 sec	3x10	3x10	3x12	3x12	3x12	3x12
	KICK-UP *tempo:* 1-1-3 | *rest:* 60 sec	3x10	3x10	3x12	3x12	3x15	3x15
DAY 3	**REPEAT DAY 1**						
DAY 4	**REPEAT DAY 2**						

	SINGLE SET	WEEK 1 *set x rep*	WEEK 2 *set x rep*	WEEK 3 *set x rep*	WEEK 4 *set x rep*	WEEK 5 *set x rep*	WEEK 6 *set x rep*
DAY 1	**STANDARD PULL-UP** *tempo:* 1-1-5 | *rest:* 75 sec	3x6	3x6	3x8	3x8	3x10	3x12
	WIDE-GRIP PULL-UP *tempo:* 1-1-5 | *rest:* 75 sec	3x4	3x5	3x6	3x7	3x8	3x9
	PIKE PRESS *tempo:* 1-1-2 | *rest:* 60 sec	3x7	3x7	3x8	3x8	3x10	3x10
	PUSH-UP *tempo:* 1-1-5 | *rest:* 75 sec	3x12	3x12	3x15	3x15	3x15	3x20
	PARALLEL GRIP PULL-UP *tempo:* 1-1-5 | *rest:* 75 sec	3x10	3x10	3x12	3x12	3x12	3x12
	WIDE PUSH-UP *tempo:* 1-1-3 | *rest:* 75 sec	3x12	3x12	3x15	3x15	3x15	3x15
	SQUAT *tempo:* 1-1-5 | *rest:* 75 sec	3x12	3x12	3x15	3x15	3x15	3x15
	SINGLE-LEG SQUAT *tempo:* 1-1-5 | *rest:* 75 sec	3x8	3x8	3x10	3x10	3x12	3x12
	FORWARD LUNGE *tempo:* 1-1-5 | *rest:* 75 sec	3x8	3x8	3x8	3x10	3x10	3x10
	CALF RAISE *tempo:* 1-1-5 | *rest:* 75 sec	3x12	3x12	3x12	3x12	3x12	3x12

DAY 2	**HANGING BICEPS CURL** tempo: 1-1-5 | rest: 75 sec	3x6	3x6	3x8	3x8	3x8	3x10
	CHAIR DIP tempo: 1-1-5 | rest: 75 sec	3x8	3x8	3x8	3x8	3x8	3x8
	DIAMOND PUSH-UP tempo: 1-1-5 | rest: 75 sec	3x8	3x8	3x10	3x10	3x10	3x12
	SHORT-RANGE PULL-UP (UPPER) tempo: 1-1-5 | rest: 75 sec	3x6	3x6	3x7	3x7	3x8	3x8
	PRESS-UP WITH PULL-UP BAR tempo: 1-1-5 | rest: 75 sec	3x6	3x6	3x7	3x7	3x8	3x8
	FLOOR DIP tempo: 1-1-5 | rest: 75 sec	3x10	3x10	3x12	3x12	3x12	3x12
	FRAME-ASSISTED SIT-UP tempo: 1-1-5 | rest: 75 sec	3x10	3x10	3x10	3x10	3x10	3x12
	STRAIGHT-LEG RAISE tempo: 1-1-5 | rest: 75 sec	3x8	3x8	3x8	3x8	3x10	3x10
	HANGING LEG CURL WITH ROTATION tempo: 1-1-5 | rest: 75 sec	3x5	3x5	3x6	3x6	3x6	3x6
	CRUNCH tempo: 1-1-5 | rest: 75 sec	3x12	3x12	3x12	3x15	3x15	3x15
DAY 3	**REPEAT DAY 1**						
DAY 4	**REPEAT DAY 2**						

	SUPERSETS	WEEK 1 set x rep	WEEK 2 set x rep	WEEK 3 set x rep	WEEK 4 set x rep	WEEK 5 set x rep	WEEK 6 set x rep
DAY 1	**1a. ALTERNATE-GRIP PULL-UP** tempo: 1-1-5 | rest: 15 sec	3x4	3x4	3x5	3x5	3x6	3x6
	1b. SQUAT tempo: 1-1-5 | rest: 30 sec	3x12	3x12	3x12	3x12	3x12	3x12
	2a. PUSH-UP tempo: 1-1-3 | rest: 10 sec	3x12	3x12	3x12	3x12	3x12	3x12
	2b. SPLIT SQUAT tempo: 1-1-5 | rest: 30 sec	3x6	3x7	3x8	3x8	3x9	3x9
	3a. PIKE PRESS tempo: 1-1-5 | rest: 15 sec	3x8	3x10	3x12	3x12	3x12	3x12
	3b. SINGLE-LEG BRIDGE tempo: 1-1-5 | rest: 30 sec	3x8	3x8	3x9	3x9	3x10	3x10
	4a. WIDE-GRIP PULL-UP tempo: 1-1-5 | rest: 15 sec	3x6	3x7	3x7	3x8	3x8	3x8
	4b. CALF RAISE tempo: 1-1-5 | rest: 30 sec	3x6	3x10	3x12	3x12	3x12	3x12
	5a. STAGGERED PUSH-UP tempo: 1-1-5 | rest: 15 sec	3x8	3x8	3x8	3x10	3x10	3x10
	5b. LEG EXTENSION tempo: 1-1-5 | rest: 30 sec	3x10	3x10	3x12	3x12	3x12	3x12

DAY 2	**1a. DIAMOND PUSH-UP** *tempo:* 1-1-5 | *rest:* 15 sec	3x10	3x10	3x12	3x12	3x12	3x12
	1b. HANGING LEG CURL *tempo:* 1-1-5 | *rest:* 30 sec	3x10	3x10	3x12	3x12	3x12	3x12
	2a. CLOSE-GRIP PULL-UP *tempo:* 1-1-5 | *rest:* 15 sec	3x6	3x7	3x8	3x8	3x8	3x8
	2b. TOTAL-BODY CRUNCH *tempo:* 1-1-5 | *rest:* 30 sec	3x8	3x10	3x10	3x10	3x12	3x12
	3a. TRICEPS PUSH-UP *tempo:* 1-1-5 | *rest:* 15 sec	3x8	3x8	3x10	3x10	3x12	3x12
	3b. ALTERNATE SINGLE-LEG RAISE *tempo:* 1-1-5 | *rest:* 30 sec	3x8	3x8	3x8	3x8	3x8	3x8
	4a. HANGING BICEPS CURL *tempo:* 1-1-5 | *rest:* 15 sec	3x7	3x8	3x8	3x8	3x10	3x10
	4b. OBLIQUE TWIST *tempo:* 1-1-5 | *rest:* 30 sec	3x6	3x7	3x7	3x8	3x8	3x8
	5a. PRESS-UP WITH PULL-UP BAR *tempo:* 1-1-5 | *rest:* 15 sec	3x6	3x7	3x7	3x8	3x8	3x8
	5b. FRAME-ASSISTED SIT-UP *tempo:* 1-1-5 | *rest:* 30 sec	3x6	3x10	3x10	3x12	3x12	3x12
DAY 3	**REPEAT DAY 1**						
DAY 4	**REPEAT DAY 2**						

MUSCULAR STRENGTH (ADVANCED)

PREREQUISITE: Muscular Strength (Intermediate) (page 68) or above average push-ups (page 37) and pull-ups (page 37)

MACROCYCLE: *Three six-week mesocycles:* Single Set (Super Slow), Supersets (Compound), Single Set (Advanced Movements). Extras: cardio 1–2 days/week. *Note:* Pay attention to the tempo of the individual exercises.

SINGLE SET	WEEK 1 set x rep	WEEK 2 set x rep	WEEK 3 set x rep	WEEK 4 set x rep	WEEK 5 set x rep	WEEK 6 set x rep
STANDARD PULL-UP *tempo:* 2-2-3 | *rest:* 60 sec	3x10	3x10	3x12	3x12	3x12	3x12
PUSH-UP *tempo:* 2-2-3 | *rest:* 60 sec	3x15	3x15	3x15	3x20	3x20	3x20
HANDSTAND SHOULDER PRESS *tempo:* 2-2-3 | *rest:* 60 sec	3x8	3x10	3x10	3x12	3x12	3x12
PARALLEL GRIP PULL-UP *tempo:* 2-2-3 | *rest:* 60 sec	3x8	3x8	3x10	3x10	3x12	3x12
STAGGERED PUSH-UP *tempo:* 2-2-3 | *rest:* 60 sec	3x6	3x6	3x7	3x7	3x8	3x8
SIDE-TO-SIDE PULL-UP *tempo:* 2-2-3 | *rest:* 60 sec	3x5	3x6	3x6	3x7	3x8	3x8
SQUAT *tempo:* 2-2-3 | *rest:* 60 sec	3x12	3x12	3x12	3x15	3x15	3x15
SINGLE-LEG BRIDGE *tempo:* 2-2-3 | *rest:* 60 sec	3x12	3x12	3x12	3x12	3x12	3x12
SPLIT SQUAT *tempo:* 2-2-3 | *rest:* 60 sec	3x10	3x10	3x10	3x12	3x12	3x12
CLOSE-GRIP PULL-UP *tempo:* 2-2-3 | *rest:* 60 sec	3x12	3x12	3x12	3x15	3x15	3x15

(DAY 1)

	Exercise	Week 1	Week 2	Week 3	Week 4	Week 5	Week 6
DAY 2	**HANGING BICEPS CURL** *tempo: 2-2-3 | rest: 60 sec*	3x15	3x15	3x20	3x20	3x25	3x25
	CHAIR DIP *tempo: 2-2-3 | rest: 60 sec*	3x10	3x10	3x12	3x12	3x15	3x15
	TRICEPS PUSH-UP *tempo: 2-2-3 | rest: 60 sec*	3x8	3x10	3x12	3x12	3x15	3x15
	CLOSE-GRIP PULL-UP *tempo: 2-2-3 | rest: 60 sec*	3x8	3x10	3x10	3x10	3x12	3x12
	PRESS-UP *tempo: 2-2-3 | rest: 60 sec*	3x8	3x8	3x10	3x12	3x12	3x12
	PIKE PRESS *tempo: 2-2-3 | rest: 60 sec*	3x12	3x12	3x12	3x12	3x15	3x15
	FRAME-ASSISTED SIT-UP *tempo: 2-2-3 | rest: 60 sec*	3x6	3x8	3x10	3x10	3x12	3x12
	STRAIGHT-LEG RAISE *tempo: 2-2-3 | rest: 60 sec*	3x10	3x10	3x10	3x12	3x12	3x12
	HANGING LEG CURL WITH ROTATION *tempo: 2-2-3 | rest: 60 sec*	3x8	3x8	3x10	3x10	3x12	3x12
	KICK-UP *tempo: 2-2-3 | rest: 60 sec*	3x8	3x8	3x10	3x10	3x12	3x12
DAY 3	**REPEAT DAY 1**						
DAY 4	**REPEAT DAY 2**						

	SUPERSETS	WEEK 1 *set x rep*	WEEK 2 *set x rep*	WEEK 3 *set x rep*	WEEK 4 *set x rep*	WEEK 5 *set x rep*	WEEK 6 *set x rep*
DAY 1	**1a. ALTERNATE-GRIP PULL-UP** *tempo: 2-2-3 | rest: 10 sec*	3x5	3x5	3x6	3x6	3x6	3x7
	1b. SQUAT *tempo: 2-2-3 | rest: 45 sec*	3x12	3x12	3x12	3x15	3x15	3x15
	2a. PUSH-UP *tempo: 2-2-3 | rest: 10 sec*	3x15	3x15	3x15	3x18	3x18	3x20
	2b. SPLIT SQUAT *tempo: 2-2-3 | rest: 45 sec*	3x10	3x10	3x12	3x12	3x12	3x12
	3a. PIKE PRESS *tempo: 2-2-3 | rest: 10 sec*	3x8	3x8	3x9	3x10	3x11	3x12
	3b. SINGLE-LEG BRIDGE *tempo: 2-2-3 | rest: 45 sec*	3x10	3x10	3x12	3x12	3x12	3x12
	4a. WIDE-GRIP PULL-UP *tempo: 2-2-3 | rest: 10 sec*	3x6	3x6	3x7	3x7	3x8	3x8
	4b. CALF RAISE *tempo: 2-2-3 | rest: 45 sec*	3x12	3x12	3x12	3x12	3x15	3x15
	5a. HANDSTAND SHOULDER PRESS *tempo: 2-2-3 | rest: 10 sec*	3x8	3x8	3x10	3x10	3x12	3x12
	5b. LEG EXTENSION *tempo: 2-2-3 | rest: 45 sec*	3x12	3x12	3x12	3x12	3x12	3x12

	1a. DIAMOND PUSH-UP *tempo:* 2-2-3 | *rest:* 10 sec	3x12	3x12	3x12	3x12	3x12	3x12
	1b. HANGING LEG CURL *tempo:* 2-2-3 | *rest:* 45 sec	3x8	3x8	3x8	3x10	3x10	3x10
	2a. CLOSE-GRIP PULL-UP *tempo:* 2-2-3 | *rest:* 10 sec	3x6	3x6	3x7	3x7	3x7	3x7
	2b. TOTAL-BODY CRUNCH *tempo:* 2-2-3 | *rest:* 45 sec	3x10	3x10	3x12	3x12	3x12	3x12
DAY 2	**3a. TRICEPS PUSH-UP** *tempo:* 2-2-3 | *rest:* 10 sec	3x10	3x10	3x10	3x10	3x12	3x12
	3b. SINGLE STRAIGHT-LEG RAISE *tempo:* 2-2-3 | *rest:* 45 sec	3x10	3x10	3x12	3x12	3x12	3x12
	4a. HANGING BICEPS CURL *tempo:* 2-2-3 | *rest:* 10 sec	3x8	3x8	3x10	3x10	3x10	3x12
	4b. HANGING LEG CURL *tempo:* 2-2-3 | *rest:* 45 sec	3x8	3x8	3x10	3x10	3x10	3x10
	5a. PRESS-UP WITH PULL-UP BAR *tempo:* 2-2-3 | *rest:* 10 sec	3x10	3x10	3x10	3x12	3x12	3x12
	5b. FRAME-ASSISTED SIT-UP *tempo:* 2-2-3 | *rest:* 45 sec	3x12	3x12	3x12	3x12	3x15	3x15
DAY 3	**REPEAT DAY 1**						
DAY 4	**REPEAT DAY 2**						

	SINGLE SET	**WEEK 1** set x rep	**WEEK 2** set x rep	**WEEK 3** set x rep	**WEEK 4** set x rep	**WEEK 5** set x rep	**WEEK 6** set x rep
	STANDARD PULL-UP *tempo:* 5-2-5 | *rest:* 60 sec	2x10	2x10	2x12	3x10	3x10	3x12
	PUSH-UP *tempo:* 5-2-5 | *rest:* 60 sec	2x15	2x15	2x15	3x15	3x15	3x15
	HANDSTAND SHOULDER PRESS *tempo:* 5-2-5 | *rest:* 60 sec	2x8	2x10	2x10	3x8	3x10	3x10
	PARALLEL GRIP PULL-UP *tempo:* 5-2-5 | *rest:* 60 sec	2x8	2x8	2x10	3x8	3x8	3x10
DAY 1	**STAGGERED PUSH-UP** *tempo:* 5-2-5 | *rest:* 60 sec	2x6	2x6	2x7	3x6	3x6	3x7
	SIDE-TO-SIDE PULL-UP *tempo:* 5-2-5 | *rest:* 60 sec	2x5	2x6	2x6	3x5	3x6	3x6
	SQUAT *tempo:* 5-2-5 | *rest:* 60 sec	2x12	2x12	2x12	3x12	3x12	3x12
	SINGLE-LEG BRIDGE *tempo:* 5-2-5 | *rest:* 60 sec	2x12	2x12	2x12	3x12	3x12	3x12
	SPLIT SQUAT *tempo:* 5-2-5 | *rest:* 60 sec	2x10	2x10	2x10	3x10	3x10	3x10
	LEG EXTENSION *tempo:* 5-2-5 | *rest:* 60 sec	2x12	2x12	2x12	3x12	3x12	3x12

DAY 2	**HANGING BICEPS CURL** *tempo:* 5-2-5 | *rest:* 60 sec	2x10	2x10	2x10	3x10	3x10	3x10
	CHAIR DIP *tempo:* 5-2-5 | *rest:* 60 sec	2x10	2x10	2x10	3x10	3x10	3x10
	TRICEPS PUSH-UP *tempo:* 5-2-5 | *rest:* 60 sec	2x12	2x12	2x12	3x12	3x12	3x12
	CLOSE-GRIP PULL-UP *tempo:* 5-2-5 | *rest:* 60 sec	2x6	2x7	2x7	3x6	3x7	3x7
	PRESS-UP *tempo:* 5-2-5 | *rest:* 60 sec	2x8	2x8	2x8	3x8	3x8	3x8
	PIKE PRESS *tempo:* 5-2-5 | *rest:* 60 sec	2x8	2x8	2x8	3x8	3x8	3x8
	FRAME-ASSISTED SIT-UP *tempo:* 5-2-5 | *rest:* 60 sec	2x10	2x10	2x10	3x10	3x10	3x10
	STRAIGHT-LEG RAISE *tempo:* 5-2-5 | *rest:* 60 sec	2x10	2x10	2x10	3x10	3x10	3x10
	HANGING LEG CURL WITH ROTATION *tempo:* 5-2-5 | *rest:* 60 sec	2x8	2x8	2x10	3x8	3x8	3x10
	KICK-UP *tempo:* 1-1-3 | *rest:* 60 sec	2x8	2x8	2x10	3x8	3x8	3x10
DAY 3	**REPEAT DAY 1**						
DAY 4	**REPEAT DAY 2**						

BODY SCULPTING (INTERMEDIATE)

PREREQUISITE: Muscular Strength (Intermediate) (page 68) or above average push-ups (page 37), chair squats (page 38) and abdominal crunches (page 38)

MACROCYCLE: *Three six-week mesocycles:* Supersets (Compound), Repetition Circuit, Modified Tabata. *Extras:* cardio 3–4 days/week, 30 min moderate to high intensity.

	SUPERSETS	WEEK 1 set x rep	WEEK 2 set x rep	WEEK 3 set x rep	WEEK 4 set x rep	WEEK 5 set x rep	WEEK 6 set x rep
DAY 1	**1a. STANDARD PULL-UP** *tempo:* 1-1-3 | *rest:* 10 sec	3x10	3x10	3x12	3x12	3x12	3x12
	1b. PUSH-UP *tempo:* 1-1-3 | *rest:* 30 sec	3x12	3x12	3x15	3x20	3x20	3x25
	2a. PARALLEL GRIP PULL-UP *tempo:* 1-1-3 | *rest:* 10 sec	3x10	3x10	3x12	3x12	3x12	3x12
	2b. DIAMOND PUSH-UP *tempo:* 1-1-2 | *rest:* 30 sec	3x8	3x8	3x10	3x10	3x10	3x12
	3a. HANGING BICEPS CURL *tempo:* 1-1-2 | *rest:* 10 sec	3x8	3x8	3x10	3x10	3x10	3x12
	3b. PRESS-UP WITH PULL-UP BAR *tempo:* 1-1-2 | *rest:* 30 sec	3x8	3x10	3x10	3x10	3x12	3x12
	4a. ALTERNATE-GRIP PUSH-UP W/BAR *tempo:* 1-1-3 | *rest:* 10 sec	3x7	3x7	3x8	3x8	3x8	3x10
	4b. SIDE-FACING PULL-UP *tempo:* 1-1-3 | *rest:* 30 sec	3x5	3x5	3x5	3x6	3x6	3x6
	5a. STANDING WALK-OUT *tempo:* 1-1-3 | *rest:* 10 sec	3x8	3x8	3x10	3x10	3x10	3x12
	5b. TRICEPS PUSH-UP *tempo:* 1-1-2 | *rest:* 30 sec	3x8	3x10	3x12	3x12	3x15	3x15

1a. SPEED SQUAT *tempo:* fast | *rest:* 10 sec	3x15	3x15	3x20	3x20	3x20	3x20
1b. LEG EXTENSION *tempo:* 1-1-2 | *rest:* 30 sec	3x15	3x15	3x1	3x20	3x20	3x20
2a. FULL CIRCLE *tempo:* 1-1-2 | *rest:* 10 sec	3x6	3x6	3x7	3x7	3x7	3x8
2b. LEG CURL *tempo:* 1-1-2 | *rest:* 30 sec	3x12	3x12	3x15	3x15	3x15	3x20
3a. FORWARD LUNGE *tempo:* 1-1-3 | *rest:* 10 sec	3x8	3x10	3x12	3x12	3x12	3x15
3b. SINGLE-LEG SQUAT *tempo:* 1-1-3 | *rest:* 30 sec	3x8	3x10	3x10	3x12	3x12	3x15
4a. HANGING BICYCLE *tempo:* 1-1-1 | *rest:* 10 sec	3x12	3x12	3x12	3x15	3x15	3x15
4b. SIDE PLANK *tempo:* 1-1-2 | *rest:* 30 sec	3x10	3x10	3x12	3x12	3x12	3x15
5a. SQUAT *tempo:* 1-1-3 | *rest:* 10 sec	3x15	3x15	3x20	3x20	3x20	3x25
5b. SINGLE-LEG BRIDGE *tempo:* 1-1-2 | *rest:* 30 sec	3x12	3x12	3x12	3x12	3x15	3x15
1a. PIKE PRESS *tempo:* 1-1-3 | *rest:* 10 sec	3x10	3x10	3x12	3x12	3x12	3x15
1b. SHOULDER TOUCH *tempo:* fast | *rest:* 30 sec	3x12	3x12	3x12	3x12	3x15	3x15
2a. PARALLEL GRIP PULL-UP *tempo:* 1-1-2 | *rest:* 10 sec	3x10	3x10	3x12	3x12	3x12	3x13
2b. ISOMETRIC HOLD (SIDE TO SIDE) *tempo:* 1-1-1 | *rest:* 30 sec	3x6	3x7	3x8	3x9	3x10	3x11
3a. BICYCLE CRUNCH *tempo:* 1-1-1 | *rest:* 10 sec	3x12	3x12	3x12	3x15	3x15	3x15
3b. PLANK *tempo:* 1-60-1 | *rest:* 30 sec	3x1	3x1	3x1	3x1	3x1	3x1
4a. SIDE-TO-SIDE PULL-UP *tempo:* 1-1-3 | *rest:* 10 sec	3x5	3x5	3x6	3x6	3x6	3x6
4b. PRESS-UP *tempo:* 1-1-2 | *rest:* 30 sec	3x10	3x10	3x12	3x12	3x12	3x12
5a. TOTAL-BODY CRUNCH *tempo:* 1-1-3 | *rest:* 10 sec	3x12	3x12	3x15	3x15	3x15	3x15
5b. SIDE PLANK *tempo:* 1-20-1 | *rest:* 30 sec	3x1	3x1	3x1	3x1	3x1	3x1

DAY 2 (rows 1a–5b, first group)

DAY 3 (rows 1a–5b, second group)

REPETITION CIRCUIT	WEEK 1 REPS	WEEK 2 REPS	WEEK 3 REPS	WEEK 4 REPS	WEEK 5 REPS	WEEK 6 REPS
STANDARD PULL-UP *tempo:* 1-1-3 | *rest:* 15 sec	10	10	12	12	15	15
STAGGERED PUSH-UP *tempo:* 1-1-3 | *rest:* 15 sec	10	10	12	12	15	15
HANGING LEG CURL *tempo:* 1-1-2 | *rest:* 15 sec	10	10	12	12	15	15
FLOOR DIP *tempo:* 1-1-2 | *rest:* 15 sec	12	12	15	15	18	18
PIKE PRESS *tempo:* 1-1-3 | *rest:* 15 sec	12	12	15	15	18	18
STANDING WALK-OUT *tempo:* 1-1-3 | *rest:* 15 sec	12	12	15	15	18	18
SIDE-TO-SIDE PULL-UP *tempo:* 1-1-3 | *rest:* 15 sec	6	6	8	8	10	10
PLANK WALK-UP *tempo:* 1-1-2 | *rest:* 15 sec	6	6	8	8	10	10
DIP WITH BAR *tempo:* 1-1-2 | *rest:* 15 sec	12	12	15	15	18	18
CRUNCH *tempo:* 1-1-2 | *rest:* 15 sec	20	20	25	25	30	30
ROUNDS	3	3	3	3	3	3
ALTERNATE-GRIP PULL-UP *tempo:* 1-1-3 | *rest:* 15 sec	6	6	8	8	10	10
PRESS-UP WITH PULL-UP BAR *tempo:* 1-1-2 | *rest:* 15 sec	10	10	12	12	15	15
SIDE PLANK *tempo:* 1-1-2 | *rest:* 15 sec	10	10	12	12	15	15
ALTERNATE SINGLE-LEG RAISE *tempo:* 1-1-3 | *rest:* 15 sec	10	10	12	12	15	15
TOTAL-BODY CRUNCH *tempo:* 1-1-2 | *rest:* 15 sec	12	12	15	15	18	18
L-SHAPED PULL-UP *tempo:* 1-1-2 | *rest:* 15 sec	10	10	12	12	15	15
POWER PUSH-UP *tempo:* fast | *rest:* 15 sec	12	12	15	15	18	18
REVERSE LUNGE *tempo:* 1-1-3 | *rest:* 15 sec	12	12	15	15	18	18
HANGING BICEPS CURL *tempo:* 1-1-2 | *rest:* 15 sec	12	12	15	15	18	18
PUSH-UP *tempo:* 1-1-1 | *rest:* 15 sec	15	15	18	18	20	20
ROUNDS	3	3	3	3	3	3

DAY 1 (rows STANDARD PULL-UP through ROUNDS)

DAY 2 (rows ALTERNATE-GRIP PULL-UP through ROUNDS)

	ISOMETRIC HOLD *tempo:* 1-1-2 | *rest:* 15 sec	10	10	12	12	15	15
	PUSH-UP *tempo:* 1-1-3 | *rest:* 15 sec	18	18	20	20	25	25
	PARALLEL GRIP PULL-UP *tempo:* 1-1-3 | *rest:* 15 sec	12	12	15	15	18	18
	SPEED SQUAT *tempo:* fast | *rest:* 15 sec	20	20	25	25	30	30
	SPLIT SQUAT *tempo:* 1-1-3 | *rest:* 15 sec	10	10	12	12	15	15
DAY 3	**PULL-UP WITH HIGH LEG RAISE** *tempo:* 1-1-3 | *rest:* 15 sec	6	6	8	8	10	10
	PLANK *tempo:* 1-60-1 | *rest:* 15 sec	1	1	1	1	1	1
	HIGH TWIST *tempo:* 1-1-2 | *rest:* 15 sec	8	8	10	10	12	12
	PRESS-UP WITH PULL-UP BAR *tempo:* 1-1-3 | *rest:* 15 sec	10	10	12	12	15	15
	CHAIR DIP *tempo:* 1-1-2 | *rest:* 15 sec	10	10	12	12	15	15
	ROUNDS	3	3	3	3	3	3

	MODIFIED TABATA	**WEEK 1** *set x duration*	**WEEK 2** *set x duration*	**WEEK 3** *set x duration*	**WEEK 4** *set x duration*	**WEEK 5** *set x duration*	**WEEK 6** *set x duration*
	1a. PUSH-UP *rest:* 10 sec	4x20 sec	4x20 sec	4x20 sec	4x20 sec	4x20 sec	4x20 sec
	1b. CLOSE-GRIP PULL-UP *rest:* 10 sec	4x20 sec	4x20 sec	4x20 sec	4x20 sec	4x20 sec	4x20 sec
	2a. PRESS-UP WITH PULL-UP BAR *rest:* 10 sec	4x20 sec	4x20 sec	4x20 sec	4x20 sec	4x20 sec	4x20 sec
	2b. HANGING BICEPS CURL *rest:* 10 sec	4x20 sec	4x20 sec	4x20 sec	4x20 sec	4x20 sec	4x20 sec
DAY 1	**3a. SQUAT** *rest:* 10 sec	4x20 sec	4x20 sec	4x20 sec	4x20 sec	4x20 sec	4x20 sec
	3b. LEG EXTENSION *rest:* 10 sec	4x20 sec	4x20 sec	4x20 sec	4x20 sec	4x20 sec	4x20 sec
	4a. HANGING LEG CURL *rest:* 10 sec	4x20 sec	4x20 sec	4x20 sec	4x20 sec	4x20 sec	4x20 sec
	4b. TOTAL-BODY CRUNCH *rest:* 10 sec	4x20 sec	4x20 sec	4x20 sec	4x20 sec	4x20 sec	4x20 sec
	5a. SHORT-RANGE PULL-UP (LOWER) *rest:* 10 sec	4x20 sec	4x20 sec	4x20 sec	4x20 sec	4x20 sec	4x20 sec
	5b. FLOOR DIP *rest:* 10 sec	4x20 sec	4x20 sec	4x20 sec	4x20 sec	4x20 sec	4x20 sec

DAY 2	**1a. CHIN-UP** rest: 10 sec	4x20 sec	4x20 sec	4x20 sec	4x20 sec	4x20 sec	4x20 sec
	1b. CHAIR DIP rest: 10 sec	4x20 sec	4x20 sec	4x20 sec	4x20 sec	4x20 sec	4x20 sec
	2a. MODIFIED PULL-UP rest: 10 sec	4x20 sec	4x20 sec	4x20 sec	4x20 sec	4x20 sec	4x20 sec
	2b. STANDING WALK-OUT rest: 10 sec	4x20 sec	4x20 sec	4x20 sec	4x20 sec	4x20 sec	4x20 sec
	3a. SPLIT SQUAT rest: 10 sec	4x20 sec	4x20 sec	4x20 sec	4x20 sec	4x20 sec	4x20 sec
	3b. SINGLE-LEG BRIDGE rest: 10 sec	4x20 sec	4x20 sec	4x20 sec	4x20 sec	4x20 sec	4x20 sec
	4a. HANGING BICYCLE rest: 10 sec	4x20 sec	4x20 sec	4x20 sec	4x20 sec	4x20 sec	4x20 sec
	4b. PLANK TO SIDE PLANK rest: 10 sec	4x20 sec	4x20 sec	4x20 sec	4x20 sec	4x20 sec	4x20 sec
	5a. DIAMOND PUSH-UP rest: 10 sec	4x20 sec	4x20 sec	4x20 sec	4x20 sec	4x20 sec	4x20 sec
	5b. DIP WITH BAR rest: 10 sec	4x20 sec	4x20 sec	4x20 sec	4x20 sec	4x20 sec	4x20 sec
DAY 3	**1a. PARALLEL GRIP PULL-UP** rest: 10 sec	4x20 sec	4x20 sec	4x20 sec	4x20 sec	4x20 sec	4x20 sec
	1b. POWER PUSH-UP rest: 10 sec	4x20 sec	4x20 sec	4x20 sec	4x20 sec	4x20 sec	4x20 sec
	2a. PRESS-UP WITH PULL-UP BAR rest: 10 sec	4x20 sec	4x20 sec	4x20 sec	4x20 sec	4x20 sec	4x20 sec
	2b. PIKE PRESS rest: 10 sec	4x20 sec	4x20 sec	4x20 sec	4x20 sec	4x20 sec	4x20 sec
	3a. REVERSE LUNGE rest: 10 sec	4x20 sec	4x20 sec	4x20 sec	4x20 sec	4x20 sec	4x20 sec
	3b. JUMPING LUNGE rest: 10 sec	4x20 sec	4x20 sec	4x20 sec	4x20 sec	4x20 sec	4x20 sec
	4a. TOTAL-BODY CRUNCH rest: 10 sec	4x20 sec	4x20 sec	4x20 sec	4x20 sec	4x20 sec	4x20 sec
	4b. FRAME-ASSISTED SIT-UP rest: 10 sec	4x20 sec	4x20 sec	4x20 sec	4x20 sec	4x20 sec	4x20 sec
	5a. PULL-UP rest: 10 sec	4x20 sec	4x20 sec	4x20 sec	4x20 sec	4x20 sec	4x20 sec
	5b. CLOSE-GRIP PULL-UP rest: 10 sec	4x20 sec	4x20 sec	4x20 sec	4x20 sec	4x20 sec	4x20 sec

CARDIO CONDITIONING (INTERMEDIATE)

PREREQUISITE: Weight Loss (Intermediate) (page 63) or above average 1.5-mile time (page 39)

MACROCYCLE: *Three six-week mesocycles:* Timed Circuit, Modified Tabata, Tabata. *Extras:* cardio 3 days/week, 20 min high intensity.

TIMED CIRCUIT	WEEK 1 duration	WEEK 2 duration	WEEK 3 duration	WEEK 4 duration	WEEK 5 duration	WEEK 6 duration
SQUAT THRUST rest: 20 sec	50 sec	50 sec	50 sec	60 sec	60 sec	60 sec
PULL-UP WITH PRESS-OUT rest: 20 sec	50 sec	50 sec	50 sec	60 sec	60 sec	60 sec
REVERSE LUNGE rest: 20 sec	50 sec	50 sec	50 sec	60 sec	60 sec	60 sec
ISOMETRIC HOLD (SIDE TO SIDE) rest: 20 sec	50 sec	50 sec	50 sec	60 sec	60 sec	60 sec
SPEED SQUAT rest: 20 sec	50 sec	50 sec	50 sec	60 sec	60 sec	60 sec
ALTERNATE SINGLE-LEG RAISE SIDE TO SIDE rest: 20 sec	50 sec	50 sec	50 sec	60 sec	60 sec	60 sec
POWER PUSH-UP rest: 20 sec	50 sec	50 sec	50 sec	60 sec	60 sec	60 sec
TOTAL-BODY CRUNCH rest: 20 sec	50 sec	50 sec	50 sec	60 sec	60 sec	60 sec
SINGLE-LEG BRIDGE rest: 20 sec	50 sec	50 sec	50 sec	60 sec	60 sec	60 sec
HIGH KNEES rest: 20 sec	50 sec	50 sec	50 sec	60 sec	60 sec	60 sec
ROUNDS	3	3	3	3	3	3
SQUAT JUMP rest: 20 sec	50 sec	50 sec	50 sec	60 sec	60 sec	60 sec
SIDE-FACING PULL-UP rest: 20 sec	50 sec	50 sec	50 sec	60 sec	60 sec	60 sec
HIGH TWIST rest: 20 sec	50 sec	50 sec	50 sec	60 sec	60 sec	60 sec
SQUAT rest: 20 sec	50 sec	50 sec	50 sec	60 sec	60 sec	60 sec
BICYCLE CRUNCH rest: 20 sec	50 sec	50 sec	50 sec	60 sec	60 sec	60 sec
SKATER rest: 20 sec	50 sec	50 sec	50 sec	60 sec	60 sec	60 sec
PLANK rest: 20 sec	50 sec	50 sec	50 sec	60 sec	60 sec	60 sec
ALTERNATE-GRIP PUSH-UP WITH BAR rest: 20 sec	50 sec	50 sec	50 sec	60 sec	60 sec	60 sec
DIP WITH BAR rest: 20 sec	50 sec	50 sec	50 sec	60 sec	60 sec	60 sec
HIGH KNEES rest: 20 sec	50 sec	50 sec	50 sec	60 sec	60 sec	60 sec
ROUNDS	3	3	3	3	3	3

DAY 1 (rows 1–11), DAY 2 (rows 12–21)

DAY 3						
MOUNTAIN CLIMBER *rest:* 20 sec	50 sec	50 sec	50 sec	60 sec	60 sec	60 sec
SPLIT SQUAT *rest:* 20 sec	50 sec	50 sec	50 sec	60 sec	60 sec	60 sec
PUSH-UP WITH ROTATION *rest:* 20 sec	50 sec	50 sec	50 sec	60 sec	60 sec	60 sec
STRAIGHT-LEG RAISE *rest:* 20 sec	50 sec	50 sec	50 sec	60 sec	60 sec	60 sec
SHOULDER TOUCH *rest:* 20 sec	50 sec	50 sec	50 sec	60 sec	60 sec	60 sec
PULL-UP WITH HIGH LEG RAISE *rest:* 20 sec	50 sec	50 sec	50 sec	60 sec	60 sec	60 sec
FRAME-ASSISTED SIT-UP *rest:* 20 sec	50 sec	50 sec	50 sec	60 sec	60 sec	60 sec
PIKE PRESS *rest:* 20 sec	50 sec	50 sec	50 sec	60 sec	60 sec	60 sec
SINGLE-LEG SQUAT *rest:* 20 sec	50 sec	50 sec	50 sec	60 sec	60 sec	60 sec
SQUAT THRUST INTO PULL-UP *rest:* 20 sec	50 sec	50 sec	50 sec	60 sec	60 sec	60 sec
ROUNDS	2	3	2	3	2	3

DAY 1 — MODIFIED TABATA	WEEK 1 set x duration	WEEK 2 set x duration	WEEK 3 set x duration	WEEK 4 set x duration	WEEK 5 set x duration	WEEK 6 set x duration
1a. HIGH KNEES *rest:* 10 sec between sets	4x20 sec	4x20 sec	4x20 sec	4x20 sec	4x20 sec	4x20 sec
1b. POWER PUSH-UP *rest:* 10 sec between sets	4x20 sec	4x20 sec	4x20 sec	4x20 sec	4x20 sec	4x20 sec
2a. SQUAT THRUST *rest:* 10 sec between sets	4x20 sec	4x20 sec	4x20 sec	4x20 sec	4x20 sec	4x20 sec
2b. DIP WITH BAR *rest:* 10 sec between sets	4x20 sec	4x20 sec	4x20 sec	4x20 sec	4x20 sec	4x20 sec
3a. SKATER *rest:* 10 sec between sets	4x20 sec	4x20 sec	4x20 sec	4x20 sec	4x20 sec	4x20 sec
3b. PULL-UP *rest:* 10 sec between sets	4x20 sec	4x20 sec	4x20 sec	4x20 sec	4x20 sec	4x20 sec
4a. SPEED SQUAT *rest:* 10 sec between sets	4x20 sec	4x20 sec	4x20 sec	4x20 sec	4x20 sec	4x20 sec
4b. FRAME-ASSISTED SIT-UP *rest:* 10 sec between sets	4x20 sec	4x20 sec	4x20 sec	4x20 sec	4x20 sec	4x20 sec

DAY 2	**1a. SQUAT JUMP** *rest:* 10 sec between sets	4x20 sec	4x20 sec	4x20 sec	4x20 sec	4x20 sec	4x20 sec
	1b. PULL-UP *rest:* 10 sec between sets	4x20 sec	4x20 sec	4x20 sec	4x20 sec	4x20 sec	4x20 sec
	2a. MOUNTAIN CLIMBER *rest:* 10 sec between sets	4x20 sec	4x20 sec	4x20 sec	4x20 sec	4x20 sec	4x20 sec
	2b. SHOULDER TOUCH *rest:* 10 sec between sets	4x20 sec	4x20 sec	4x20 sec	4x20 sec	4x20 sec	4x20 sec
	3a. HANGING BICEPS CURL *rest:* 10 sec between sets	4x20 sec	4x20 sec	4x20 sec	4x20 sec	4x20 sec	4x20 sec
	3b. JUMPING LUNGE *rest:* 10 sec between sets	4x20 sec	4x20 sec	4x20 sec	4x20 sec	4x20 sec	4x20 sec
	4a. TOTAL-BODY CRUNCH *rest:* 10 sec between sets	4x20 sec	4x20 sec	4x20 sec	4x20 sec	4x20 sec	4x20 sec
	4b. SPEED SQUAT *rest:* 10 sec between sets	4x20 sec	4x20 sec	4x20 sec	4x20 sec	4x20 sec	4x20 sec
DAY 3	**1a. SQUAT THRUST** *rest:* 10 sec between sets	4x20 sec	4x20 sec	4x20 sec	4x20 sec	4x20 sec	4x20 sec
	1b. HIGH TWIST *rest:* 10 sec between sets	4x20 sec	4x20 sec	4x20 sec	4x20 sec	4x20 sec	4x20 sec
	2a. CHIN-UP *rest:* 10 sec between sets	4x20 sec	4x20 sec	4x20 sec	4x20 sec	4x20 sec	4x20 sec
	2b. MOUNTAIN CLIMBER *rest:* 10 sec between sets	4x20 sec	4x20 sec	4x20 sec	4x20 sec	4x20 sec	4x20 sec
	3a. HIGH KNEES *rest:* 10 sec between sets	4x20 sec	4x20 sec	4x20 sec	4x20 sec	4x20 sec	4x20 sec
	3b. STAGGERED PUSH-UP *rest:* 10 sec between sets	4x20 sec	4x20 sec	4x20 sec	4x20 sec	4x20 sec	4x20 sec
	4a. SQUAT JUMP *rest:* 10 sec between sets	4x20 sec	4x20 sec	4x20 sec	4x20 sec	4x20 sec	4x20 sec
	4b. CHAIR DIP *rest:* 10 sec between sets	4x20 sec	4x20 sec	4x20 sec	4x20 sec	4x20 sec	4x20 sec

TABATA	WEEK 1 set x duration	WEEK 2 set x duration	WEEK 3 set x duration	WEEK 4 set x duration	WEEK 5 set x duration	WEEK 6 set x duration
SQUAT JUMP *rest:* 10 sec between sets	4x20 sec	4x20 sec	4x20 sec	4x20 sec	4x20 sec	4x20 sec
PUSH-UP *rest:* 10 sec between sets	4x20 sec	4x20 sec	4x20 sec	4x20 sec	4x20 sec	4x20 sec
BICYCLE CRUNCH *rest:* 10 sec between sets	4x20 sec	4x20 sec	4x20 sec	4x20 sec	4x20 sec	4x20 sec
HANGING LEG CURL *rest:* 10 sec between sets	4x20 sec	4x20 sec	4x20 sec	4x20 sec	4x20 sec	4x20 sec
SHOULDER TOUCH *rest:* 10 sec between sets	4x20 sec	4x20 sec	4x20 sec	4x20 sec	4x20 sec	4x20 sec
HIGH KNEES *rest:* 10 sec between sets	4x20 sec	4x20 sec	4x20 sec	4x20 sec	4x20 sec	4x20 sec
HANGING BICEPS CURL *rest:* 10 sec between sets	4x20 sec	4x20 sec	4x20 sec	4x20 sec	4x20 sec	4x20 sec
SPEED SQUAT *rest:* 10 sec between sets	4x20 sec	4x20 sec	4x20 sec	4x20 sec	4x20 sec	4x20 sec
CHIN-UP *rest:* 10 sec between sets	4x20 sec	4x20 sec	4x20 sec	4x20 sec	4x20 sec	4x20 sec
FRAME-ASSISTED SIT-UP *rest:* 10 sec between sets	4x20 sec	4x20 sec	4x20 sec	4x20 sec	4x20 sec	4x20 sec
MOUNTAIN CLIMBER *rest:* 10 sec between sets	4x20 sec	4x20 sec	4x20 sec	4x20 sec	4x20 sec	4x20 sec
OBLIQUE TWIST *rest:* 10 sec between sets	4x20 sec	4x20 sec	4x20 sec	4x20 sec	4x20 sec	4x20 sec
JUMPING LUNGE *rest:* 10 sec between sets	4x20 sec	4x20 sec	4x20 sec	4x20 sec	4x20 sec	4x20 sec
DIP WITH BAR *rest:* 10 sec between sets	4x20 sec	4x20 sec	4x20 sec	4x20 sec	4x20 sec	4x20 sec
ALTERNATE-GRIP PULL-UP *rest:* 10 sec between sets	4x20 sec	4x20 sec	4x20 sec	4x20 sec	4x20 sec	4x20 sec

(DAY 1: Squat Jump, Push-Up, Bicycle Crunch, Hanging Leg Curl, Shoulder Touch)
(DAY 2: High Knees, Hanging Biceps Curl, Speed Squat, Chin-Up, Frame-Assisted Sit-Up)
(DAY 3: Mountain Climber, Oblique Twist, Jumping Lunge, Dip with Bar, Alternate-Grip Pull-Up)

CARDIO CONDITIONING (ADVANCED)

PREREQUISITE: Cardio Conditioning (Intermediate) (page 81) or above average 1.5-mile run (page 39), push-ups (page 37), pull-ups (page 37) and 25+ squat thrusts

MACROCYCLE: *Three six-week mesocycles:* Trisets (each triset begins with a cardio exercise), Timed Circuit, Tabata. *Extras:* cardio 3–5 days/week, alternating moderate-intensity long-duration and high-intensity short-duration cardio.

TRISETS	WEEK 1 *set x rep*	WEEK 2 *set x rep*	WEEK 3 *set x rep*	WEEK 4 *set x rep*	WEEK 5 *set x rep*	WEEK 6 *set x rep*
1a. HIGH KNEES *tempo:* fast | *rest:* 5 sec	3x60 sec	3x60 sec	3x60 sec	3x60 sec	3x75 sec	3x75 sec
1b. TOTAL BODY EXPLOSIVE PUSH-UP *tempo:* fast | *rest:* 5 sec	3x10	3x10	3x12	3x12	3x12	3x15
1c. TOTAL-BODY CRUNCH *tempo:* 1-1-2 | *rest:* 15 sec	3x12	3x12	3x15	3x15	3x20	3x20
2a. SQUAT THRUST *tempo:* fast | *rest:* 5 sec	3x60 sec	3x60 sec	3x60 sec	3x60 sec	3x75 sec	3x75 sec
2b. STANDARD PULL-UP *tempo:* 1-1-3 | *rest:* 5 sec	3x12	3x12	3x15	3x15	3x18	3x20
2c. REVERSE LUNGE *tempo:* 1-1-2 | *rest:* 15 sec	3x10	3x10	3x12	3x12	3x12	3x12
3a. SKATER *tempo:* fast | *rest:* 5 sec	3x60 sec	3x60 sec	3x60 sec	3x60 sec	3x75 sec	3x75 sec
3b. PULL-UP WITH PRESS-OUT *tempo:* 1-1-3 | *rest:* 5 sec	3x12	3x12	3x12	3x12	3x12	3x12
3c. PLANK WITH ARM EXTENSION *tempo:* 1-1-1 | *rest:* 15 sec	3x15	3x15	3x15	3x15	3x15	3x15
4a. SQUAT JUMP *tempo:* fast | *rest:* 5 sec	3x60 sec	3x60 sec	3x60 sec	3x60 sec	3x75 sec	3x75 sec
4b. PRESS-UP *tempo:* 1-1-2 | *rest:* 5 sec	3x12	3x12	3x12	3x15	3x15	3x15
4c. HALF CIRCLE *tempo:* 1-1-3 | *rest:* 15 sec	3x12	3x12	3x12	3x12	3x12	3x12
5a. JUMPING LUNGE *tempo:* fast | *rest:* 5 sec	3x60 sec	3x60 sec	3x60 sec	3x60 sec	3x75 sec	3x75 sec
5b. ISOMETRIC HOLD *tempo:* 1-20-1 | *rest:* 5 sec	3x20 sec	3x20 sec	3x20 sec	3x20 sec	3x20 sec	3x20 sec
5c. STRAIGHT-LEG RAISE *tempo:* 1-1-3 | *rest:* 15 sec	3x12	3x12	3x12	3x12	3x12	3x12

DAY 1

1a. MOUNTAIN CLIMBER *tempo:* fast | *rest:* 5 sec	3x60 sec	3x60 sec	3x60 sec	3x60 sec	3x60 sec	3x60 sec
1b. ISOMETRIC HOLD (SIDE TO SIDE) *tempo:* 1-1-1 | *rest:* 5 sec	3x12	3x12	3x15	3x15	3x15	3x15
1c. SINGLE-LEG SQUAT *tempo:* 1-1-2 | *rest:* 5 sec	3x10	3x10	3x12	3x12	3x12	3x15
2a. SHOULDER TOUCH *tempo:* fast | *rest:* 5 sec	3x60 sec	3x60 sec	3x60 sec	3x60 sec	3x60 sec	3x60 sec
2b. PULL-UP WITH HIGH LEG RAISE *tempo:* 1-1-2 | *rest:* 5 sec	3x12	3x12	3x12	3x15	3x15	3x15
2C. SIDE PLANK *tempo:* 1-1-2 | *rest:* 15 sec	3x12	3x12	3x12	3x15	3x15	3x15
3a. SQUAT THRUST *tempo:* fast | *rest:* 5 sec	3x60 sec	3x60 sec	3x60 sec	3x60 sec	3x60 sec	3x60 sec
3b. PIKE PRESS *tempo:* 1-1-2 | *rest:* 5 sec	3x8	3x10	3x12	3x15	3x15	3x20
3c. CORE WALK-OUT *tempo:* 1-1-3 | *rest:* 15 sec	3x12	3x12	3x12	3x15	3x15	3x15
4a. JUMPING LUNGE *tempo:* fast | *rest:* 5 sec	3x60 sec	3x60 sec	3x60 sec	3x60 sec	3x60 sec	3x60 sec
4b. SIDE-FACING PULL-UP *tempo:* 1-1-2 | *rest:* 5 sec	3x8	3x8	3x8	3x10	3x10	3x10
4c. HANGING OBLIQUE CRUNCH *tempo:* 1-1-2 | *rest:* 15 sec	3x8	3x8	3x8	3x10	3x10	3x10
5a. SPEED SQUAT *tempo:* fast | *rest:* 5 sec	3x60 sec	3x60 sec	3x60 sec	3x60 sec	3x60 sec	3x60 sec
5b. DIP WITH BAR *tempo:* 1-1-2 | *rest:* 5 sec	3x12	3x12	3x12	3x15	3x15	3x15
5c. BICYCLE CRUNCH *tempo:* 1-1-1 | *rest:* 15 sec	3x12	3x15	3x15	3x15	3x15	3x15

DAY 3							
1a. SQUAT THRUST INTO PULL-UP *tempo:* fast | *rest:* 5 sec	3x60 sec	3x60 sec	3x60 sec	3x60 sec	3x60 sec	3x60 sec
1b. HANDSTAND SHOULDER PRESS *tempo:* 1-1-2 | *rest:* 5 sec	3x8	3x10	3x10	3x12	3x12	3x12
1c. CRUNCH *tempo:* 1-1-2 | *rest:* 15 sec	3x25	3x25	3x25	3x25	3x25	3x30
2a. SQUAT JUMP *tempo:* fast | *rest:* 5 sec	3x60 sec	3x60 sec	3x60 sec	3x60 sec	3x60 sec	3x60 sec
2b. STAGGERED PUSH-UP *tempo:* 1-1-2 | *rest:* 5 sec	3x10	3x12	3x12	3x12	3x12	3x15
2C. FRAME-ASSISTED SIT-UP *tempo:* 1-1-2 | *rest:* 15 sec	3x15	3x15	3x15	3x20	3x20	3x20
3a. MOUNTAIN CLIMBER *tempo:* fast | *rest:* 5 sec	3x60 sec	3x60 sec	3x60 sec	3x60 sec	3x60 sec	3x60 sec
3b. PRESS-UP *tempo:* 1-1-2 | *rest:* 5 sec	3x15	3x15	3x15	3x15	3x20	3x20
3c. OBLIQUE TWIST *tempo:* 1-1-2 | *rest:* 15 sec	3x12	3x12	3x12	3x15	3x15	3x15
4a. SHOULDER TOUCH *tempo:* fast | *rest:* 5 sec	3x60 sec	3x60 sec	3x60 sec	3x60 sec	3x60 sec	3x60 sec
4b. HANGING BICEPS CURL *tempo:* 1-1-2 | *rest:* 5 sec	3x12	3x12	3x15	3x15	3x15	3x15
4c. HALF CIRCLE *tempo:* 1-1-3 | *rest:* 15 sec	3x8	3x8	3x10	3x12	3x12	3x12
5a. HIGH KNEES *tempo:* fast | *rest:* 5 sec	3x60 sec	3x60 sec	3x60 sec	3x60 sec	3x60 sec	3x60 sec
5b. PUSH-UP *tempo:* 1-1-2 | *rest:* 5 sec	3x25	3x25	3x25	3x30	3x35	3x40
5c. SPEED SQUAT *tempo:* fast | *rest:* 15 sec	3x20	3x20	3x20	3x25	3x25	3x30

	TIMED CIRCUIT	WEEK 1 duration	WEEK 2 duration	WEEK 3 duration	WEEK 4 duration	WEEK 5 duration	WEEK 6 duration
DAY 1	**HIGH KNEES** rest: 10 sec	65 sec	65 sec	75 sec	75 sec	80 sec	90 sec
	STANDARD PULL-UP rest: 10 sec	65 sec	65 sec	75 sec	75 sec	80 sec	90 sec
	SPLIT SQUAT rest: 10 sec	65 sec	65 sec	75 sec	75 sec	80 sec	90 sec
	PIKE PRESS rest: 10 sec	65 sec	65 sec	75 sec	75 sec	80 sec	90 sec
	MOUNTAIN CLIMBER rest: 10 sec	65 sec	65 sec	75 sec	75 sec	80 sec	90 sec
	OBLIQUE TWIST rest: 10 sec	65 sec	65 sec	75 sec	75 sec	80 sec	90 sec
	SHOULDER TOUCH rest: 10 sec	65 sec	65 sec	75 sec	75 sec	80 sec	90 sec
	PARALLEL GRIP PULL-UP rest: 10 sec	65 sec	65 sec	75 sec	75 sec	80 sec	90 sec
	TOTAL-BODY CRUNCH rest: 10 sec	65 sec	65 sec	75 sec	75 sec	80 sec	90 sec
	SQUAT JUMP rest: 10 sec	65 sec	65 sec	75 sec	75 sec	80 sec	90 sec
	ROUNDS	3	3	2	3	2	3
DAY 2	**SQUAT THRUST** rest: 10 sec	65 sec	65 sec	75 sec	75 sec	80 sec	90 sec
	PARALLEL GRIP PULL-UP rest: 10 sec	65 sec	65 sec	75 sec	75 sec	80 sec	90 sec
	SINGLE-LEG SQUAT rest: 10 sec	65 sec	65 sec	75 sec	75 sec	80 sec	90 sec
	SPEED SQUAT rest: 10 sec	65 sec	65 sec	75 sec	75 sec	80 sec	90 sec
	PRESS-UP rest: 10 sec	65 sec	65 sec	75 sec	75 sec	80 sec	90 sec
	SKATER rest: 10 sec	65 sec	65 sec	75 sec	75 sec	80 sec	90 sec
	HANGING LEG CURL rest: 10 sec	65 sec	65 sec	75 sec	75 sec	80 sec	90 sec
	TOTAL-BODY EXPLOSIVE PUSH-UP rest: 10 sec	65 sec	65 sec	75 sec	75 sec	80 sec	90 sec
	DIP WITH BAR rest: 10 sec	65 sec	65 sec	75 sec	75 sec	80 sec	90 sec
	JUMPING LUNGE rest: 10 sec	65 sec	65 sec	75 sec	75 sec	80 sec	90 sec
	ROUNDS	3	3	2	3	2	3
DAY 3	**REPEAT DAY 1**						
DAY 4	**REPEAT DAY 2**						

TABATA		WEEK 1 set x duration	WEEK 2 set x duration	WEEK 3 set x duration	WEEK 4 set x duration	WEEK 5 set x duration	WEEK 6 set x duration
DAY 1	**SPEED SQUAT** *rest:* 10 sec between sets	4x20 sec	4x20 sec	4x20 sec	4x20 sec	4x20 sec	4x20 sec
	PUSH-UP *rest:* 10 sec between sets	4x20 sec	4x20 sec	4x20 sec	4x20 sec	4x20 sec	4x20 sec
	SHOULDER TOUCH *rest:* 10 sec between sets	4x20 sec	4x20 sec	4x20 sec	4x20 sec	4x20 sec	4x20 sec
	PARALLEL GRIP PULL-UP *rest:* 10 sec between sets	4x20 sec	4x20 sec	4x20 sec	4x20 sec	4x20 sec	4x20 sec
	MOUNTAIN CLIMBER *rest:* 10 sec between sets	4x20 sec	4x20 sec	4x20 sec	4x20 sec	4x20 sec	4x20 sec
DAY 2	**HANGING BICEPS CURL** *rest:* 10 sec between sets	4x20 sec	4x20 sec	4x20 sec	4x20 sec	4x20 sec	4x20 sec
	SQUAT THRUST *rest:* 10 sec between sets	4x20 sec	4x20 sec	4x20 sec	4x20 sec	4x20 sec	4x20 sec
	DIP WITH BAR *rest:* 10 sec between sets	4x20 sec	4x20 sec	4x20 sec	4x20 sec	4x20 sec	4x20 sec
	JUMPING LUNGE *rest:* 10 sec between sets	4x20 sec	4x20 sec	4x20 sec	4x20 sec	4x20 sec	4x20 sec
	PIKE PRESS *rest:* 10 sec between sets	4x20 sec	4x20 sec	4x20 sec	4x20 sec	4x20 sec	4x20 sec
DAY 3	**SQUAT JUMP** *rest:* 10 sec between sets	4x20 sec	4x20 sec	4x20 sec	4x20 sec	4x20 sec	4x20 sec
	PARALLEL GRIP PULL-UP *rest:* 10 sec between sets	4x20 sec	4x20 sec	4x20 sec	4x20 sec	4x20 sec	4x20 sec
	BICYCLE CRUNCH *rest:* 10 sec between sets	4x20 sec	4x20 sec	4x20 sec	4x20 sec	4x20 sec	4x20 sec
	STAGGERED PUSH-UP *rest:* 10 sec between sets	4x20 sec	4x20 sec	4x20 sec	4x20 sec	4x20 sec	4x20 sec
	HIGH KNEES *rest:* 10 sec between sets	4x20 sec	4x20 sec	4x20 sec	4x20 sec	4x20 sec	4x20 sec

PULL-UP DEVELOPMENT PROGRAM

Depending on your pull-up assessment results, you may need to begin a program to help develop the movement. Please begin with the appropriate program. This should be in addition to your normal exercise routine.

LEVEL 1		WEEK 1 set x rep	WEEK 2 set x rep	WEEK 3 set x rep	WEEK 4 set x rep	WEEK 5 set x rep	WEEK 6 set x rep
DAY 1	**SCAPULAR PULL-UP** *tempo:* 1-2-3 | *rest:* 45 sec	3x8	3x8	3x10	3x10	3x10	3x10
	MODIFIED PULL-UP *tempo:* 1-2-3 | *rest:* 45 sec	3x8	3x8	3x10	3x10	3x12	3x12
	ISOMETRIC HOLD *tempo:* 1-10-3 | *rest:* 45 sec	2x1	2x1	2x1	2x1	2x1	2x1
	PULL-UP WITH NEGATIVE FOCUS *tempo:* 1-2-6 | *rest:* 45 sec	2x3	2x4	2x5	2x5	2x5	2x6
	SHORT-RANGE PULL-UP (UPPER) *tempo:* 1-1-3 | *rest:* 45 sec	2x3	2x3	2x4	2x5	2x6	2x7
DAY 2	**STANDARD PULL-UP** *tempo:* 1-2-3 | *rest:* 45 sec	0	2x1	3x1	3x2	3x2	3x3
	CHIN-UP *tempo:* 1-2-3 | *rest:* 45 sec	2x2	2x3	3x4	3x4	3x5	3x5
	CHAIR-ASSISTED PULL-UP *tempo:* 1-2-3 | *rest:* 45 sec	2x5	3x5	3x5	3x6	3x6	3x6
	PARTNER-ASSISTED PULL-UP *tempo:* 1-2-3 | *rest:* 60 sec	2x5	3x5	3x5	3x6	3x6	3x6
	JUMPING PULL-UP (FEET ON FLOOR) *tempo:* 1-2-3 | *rest:* 45 sec	2x5	3x5	3x5	3x5	3x5	3x5

LEVEL 2		WEEK 1 set x rep	WEEK 2 set x rep	WEEK 3 set x rep	WEEK 4 set x rep	WEEK 5 set x rep	WEEK 6 set x rep
DAY 1	**PULL-UP WITH NEGATIVE FOCUS** *tempo:* 1-2-6 | *rest:* 90 sec	2x3	2x3	2x3	2x4	2x4	2x4
	SHORT-RANGE PULL-UP (LOWER) *tempo:* 1-1-2 | *rest:* 60 sec	2x5	2x5	2x6	2x6	2x7	2x7
	SHORT-RANGE PULL-UP (UPPER) *tempo:* 1-1-2 | *rest:* 60 sec	2x4	2x4	2x5	2x5	2x6	2x6
	CHAIR-ASSISTED PULL-UP *tempo:* 1-2-3 | *rest:* 60 sec	3x6	3x6	3x7	3x7	3x8	3x9
DAY 2	**PARALLEL GRIP PULL-UP** *tempo:* 1-1-3 | *rest:* 60 sec	3x3	3x3	3x4	3x4	3x4	3x5
	JUMPING PULL-UP *tempo:* 1-1-3 | *rest:* 60 sec	2x5	2x6	2x6	2x7	2x7	2x8
	BAND-ASSISTED PULL-UP *tempo:* 1-2-3 | *rest:* 60 sec	2x6	2x7	2x7	2x8	2x8	2x8
	PARTNER-ASSISTED PULL-UP *tempo:* 1-2-3 | *rest:* 60 sec	3x8	3x8	3x9	3x9	3x9	3x10
	ISOMETRIC HOLD *tempo:* 1-12-1 | *rest:* 90 sec	2x1	2x1	2x1	2x1	2x1	2x1

LEVEL 3		WEEK 1 set x rep	WEEK 2 set x rep	WEEK 3 set x rep	WEEK 4 set x rep	WEEK 5 set x rep	WEEK 6 set x rep
DAY 1	**STANDARD PULL-UP** *tempo*: 1-1-3 | *rest*: 60 sec	3x7	3x8	3x8	3x8	3x10	3x11
	PULL-UP WITH NEGATIVE FOCUS *tempo*: 1-1-3 | *rest*: 90 sec	3x5	3x5	3x6	3x6	3x7	3x6
	PARALLEL GRIP PULL-UP *tempo*: 1-1-3 | *rest*: 60 sec	3x8	3x8	3x10	3x11	3x11	3x12
	CHIN-UP *tempo*: 1-1-3 | *rest*: 60 sec	3x8	3x8	3x10	3x10	3x11	3x12
	ALTERNATE-GRIP PULL-UP *tempo*: 1-1-3 | *rest*: 60 sec	3x5	3x5	3x6	3x6	3x7	3x7
DAY 2	**REPEAT DAY 1**						

QUICK ATHLETE'S WORKOUT

This high-intensity workout is great for conditioning and will be a challenge for any level of athlete. To modify, cut all of the numbers in half.

QUICK ATHLETE'S WORKOUT	
EXERCISE	**DURATION**
JUMP ROPE	10 minutes
STANDARD PULL-UP	15–20 reps
TOTAL-BODY CRUNCH	25 reps
PUSH-UP	100 reps
CRUNCH	100 reps
SQUAT	100 reps
SQUAT THRUST	three 1-minute rounds with 1-minute rest between rounds
HIGH KNEES	Tabata
TOTAL-BODY EXPLOSIVE PUSH-UP	20 reps

5-MINUTE EXPRESS WORKOUT (BEGINNER/INTERMEDIATE)

This complete and total-body workout can be completed in under 5 minutes.

5-MINUTE EXPRESS WORKOUT (BEGINNER/INTERMEDIATE)	
EXERCISE	DURATION
HIGH KNEES	1 min
PULL-UP	To exhaustion
PUSH-UP	15 reps
CRUNCH	15 reps
SQUAT	15 reps
PLANK	1 min
PULL-UP	To exhaustion
FULL CIRCLE	2 sets x 10 reps
HANGING LEG RAISE	Hold for 30 sec

5-MINUTE EXPRESS WORKOUT (ADVANCED)

This advanced, high-intensity, total-body workout can be completed in under 5 minutes.

5-MINUTE EXPRESS WORKOUT (ADVANCED)	
EXERCISE	DURATION
MOUNTAIN CLIMBER	1 min
PULL-UP	To exhaustion
PUSH-UP	25 reps
CRUNCH	25 reps
SQUAT	25 reps
PLANK	1 min
SQUAT THRUST	50

PART III
EXERCISES

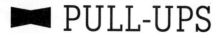 # PULL-UPS

This section covers the standard pull-up as well as its many variations. For the most part these exercises are listed progressively, meaning that we begin with the easier variations and progress to the more difficult ones. This makes choosing new exercises straightforward as you can simply pick the next exercise on the list.

TECHNIQUE

Most of the technique for pull-ups and their variations apply across the board unless otherwise noted. The following is what you need to know to perform a proper pull-up.

HAND POSITION/GRIP: There are a few different ways to position your hands for pull-ups. Each grip changes how much emphasis is placed on the lats, biceps, forearms and upper back. A chin-up (palms facing you), for example, will get more assistance from the biceps than a wide-grip pull-up. Regardless of the hand position, your grip should be secure. There isn't a huge difference between a closed loop (thumb wrapped completely around the bar) and an open loop. The open loop is slightly harder and you're prone to slipping if the bar is slippery or if your palms are sweaty, so be careful.

ARM POSITION: Ideally, your arms should be almost fully extended at the start of a pull-up. You should have a very slight bend at the elbows (it can be dangerous to be completely locked out). Return to this position after each successive repetition. The range of motion can be modified, so if you have a hard time with the full range, it's OK to shorten it.

HEAD AND NECK POSITION: Keep your head position as neutral as possible. Avoid excessively tilting your neck back or forward. Ideally, you should be facing straight ahead or tilted back slightly in order to see the bar.

SHOULDER POSITION: The scapulae (shoulder blades) are very important when performing a pull-up. Whenever you start the movement, you should first squeeze the shoulder blades together. At first, it may be necessary to isolate this movement, meaning that you'll need to squeeze the shoulder blades together and pause, followed by the rest of the pull-up. Eventually, you should be able to seamlessly transition from squeezing the shoulder blades together into the rest of the pull-up without a pause.

TORSO POSITION: Your torso should remain stable throughout. Brace the core and avoid swinging. Your spine should be neutral or with a slight arch, but avoid arching excessively.

LEG POSITION: Your feet should be off the floor when you start the movement. If your feet touch the floor when your arms are fully extended, bend your knees behind you.

GETTING TO THE BAR

If you can't reach the bar while standing on the floor, there are two options available in order to get to it.

OPTION 1: *Use a step, bench or chair.* Exercise caution and make sure that whatever you use is sturdy and level. Make sure that the step allows you to grip the bar without jumping. Place the chair or step below the bar, then step on the chair or step and make sure that it's stable. Grip the handles and bend your knees behind you.

OPTION 2: *Jump.* If the bar is within a couple of inches, extend your arms and place them in the position you'd like to grab. Go into a quarter squat and jump. It's not recommended for beginners to jump and grab more than a few inches, but if you're going to, make sure it's as safe as possible. In this case, you'll have to perform a jumping pull-up (as described on page 120) while simultaneously grabbing the bar with both arms. When doing this, make sure to stabilize your body upon grabbing the bar and slowly lowering to the starting position.

MOVEMENT

Make sure that the movement isn't herky-jerky. It should be as smooth and fluid as possible. The concentric phase (pulling up) should last 1–2 seconds. This should be followed by a 1-second pause at the top. The eccentric phase (lowering) should last 2–3 seconds and should be controlled the entire way.

TILTING THE BODY

It's normal to tilt the torso slightly at an angle when performing a pull-up. When doing this, make sure that your torso is stable — brace your core and avoid excessively arching your back.

BREATHING

Exhale as you pull yourself up, inhale as you lower yourself back to the starting position.

COMMON PROBLEMS

Excessive swinging is very common. *Solution:* Try slowing down. The slower you move, the more control you'll have over the movement. Also, shorten your range of motion temporarily. You also may have **trouble maintaining the grip**. *Solution:* Try isometric holds of up to 30 seconds.

◼ CHIN-UP

PRIMARY MUSCLES: Lats, biceps   **SECONDARY MUSCLES:** Upper back

STARTING POSITION: Grip the bar with your hands about 6–8 inches apart and palms facing you. Fully extend your arms and bend your knees in order to pick your feet off the floor.

1: Initiate the movement by squeezing your shoulder blades together and pulling yourself up until your chin is over the bar. Your arms should stay close to your body the entire way up.

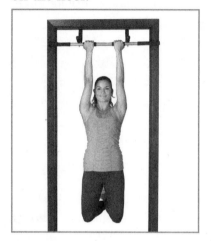

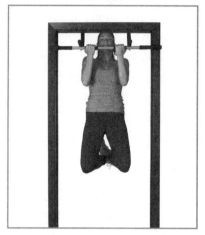

Control yourself back to the starting position. Avoid the tendency to shorten the range on the way down. Extend your arms as much as is comfortable.

◤ PARALLEL GRIP PULL-UP

PRIMARY MUSCLES: Lats, upper back   **SECONDARY MUSCLES:** Biceps

STARTING POSITION: Grip the parallel bars with your palms facing each other. Your arms should be fully extended and your legs should be off the floor.

1: Initiate the movement by squeezing your shoulder blades together and pulling yourself up until your chin is over the bar.

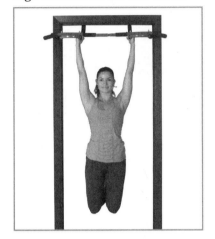

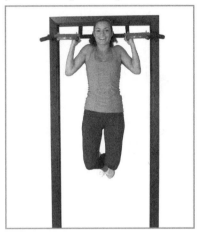

Control back down until your elbows are almost fully extended. Make sure to maintain control and stability on the way back down.

MODIFICATION: If you have trouble with this, work on a static hold.

PROGRESSION: Straighten out your legs so that your entire body is parallel to the floor.

◪ STANDARD PULL-UP

PRIMARY MUSCLES: Lats   **SECONDARY MUSCLES:** Upper back, biceps

STARTING POSITION: Grip the bar with your palms facing away from you. Your hands should be slightly wider than your shoulders. Fully extend your arms and bend your knees in order to pick your feet off the floor.

1: Initiate the movement by squeezing your shoulder blades together and pulling yourself up until your chest is close to the bar.

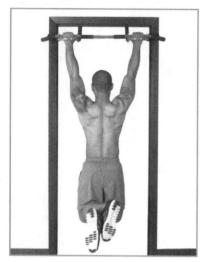

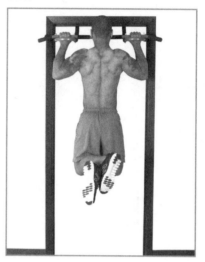

Control back down until your elbows are almost fully extended. While you may need to tilt back slightly, avoid overarching your back.

◨ ALTERNATE-GRIP PULL-UP

PRIMARY MUSCLES: Lats, biceps, forearms   **SECONDARY MUSCLES:** Upper back

STARTING POSITION: Grip the bar with your hands about shoulder-width apart. One hand should have the palm facing you and the other should have the palm facing away. Begin with both arms close to fully extended. Bend your knees in order to pick your feet off the floor.

1: Initiate the movement by squeezing your shoulder blades together and pulling yourself up until your chin is above the bar. Your arms should be close to your body.

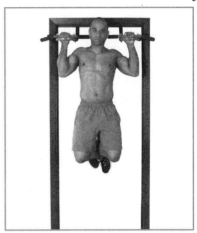

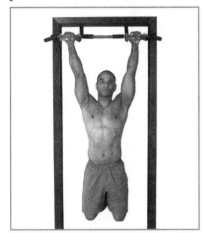

Control yourself back to the starting position.

Make sure to switch hand position. You can do this in the middle of your set or in between each set.

◼ CLOSE-GRIP PULL-UP

PRIMARY MUSCLES: Lats, forearms   **SECONDARY MUSCLES:** Upper back, biceps

STARTING POSITION: Grip the bar with your hands about 6–8 inches apart and your palms facing away from you.

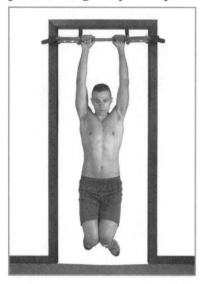

1: Initiate the movement by squeezing your shoulder blades together and pulling yourself up until your chin is above the bar. Your arms should stay close to your torso the entire way up.

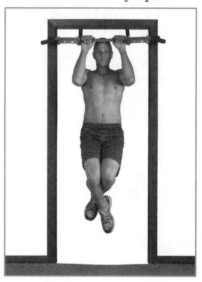

Slowly return to your starting position. Make sure to maintain a strong grip on the bar.

◪ WIDE-GRIP PULL-UP

This is a great progression on the traditional pull-up. Much of the biceps assistance is eliminated, making it much more difficult. Always do this pull-up with your hands slightly in front of your chest—never behind.

PRIMARY MUSCLES: Lats   **SECONDARY MUSCLES:** Upper back, biceps

STARTING POSITION: Grip the bar as wide as you comfortably can. Your arms should be close to fully extended with your knees bent and feet behind you.

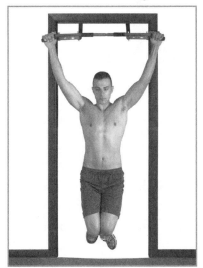

1: Initiate the movement by squeezing your shoulder blades together and pulling yourself up until your chest is within a few inches of the bar. Make sure not to overarch your back on the way up.

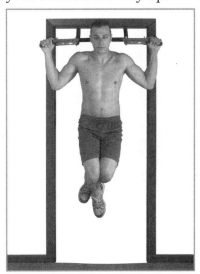

Control yourself back to starting position.

SIDE-FACING PULL-UP

PRIMARY MUSCLES: Lats, biceps   **SECONDARY MUSCLES:** Upper back

STARTING POSITION: Step underneath the bar so that your torso is perpendicular to the bar. Grip the bar as if you were holding a baseball bat, with one hand directly behind the other. Your arms should be almost fully extended with your knees bent and feet behind you.

1: Initiate the movement by squeezing your shoulder blades together and pulling yourself up. As you near the top of the movement, move your head to one side of the bar until your chin is above the bar.

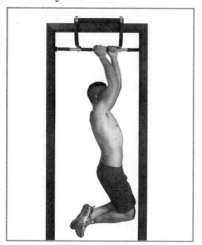

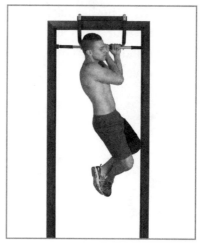

2: Slowly lower back to starting position. You can focus on keeping your head on one side of the bar per set or alternate sides within each set.

> **PROGRESSION:** At the top of the movement, lift your torso so that it's parallel to the floor.

SIDE-TO-SIDE PULL-UP

This can be done with any hand position, not just the standard pull-up grip.

PRIMARY MUSCLES: Lats, biceps   **SECONDARY MUSCLES:** Upper back

STARTING POSITION: Grip the bar with your hands slightly wider than your shoulders. Your arms should be close to fully extended with your knees bent and feet behind you.

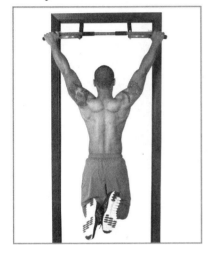

1: Pull yourself up to one side of the bar until your chin is close to the hand on the side that you're pulling up to.

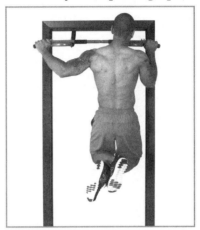

Slowly lower yourself back to starting position. You can pull yourself up to the other side and continue alternating, or complete all the reps for one side before performing the other.

PROGRESSION: Focus on one arm. If you're pulling to your right, for example, focus all of your energy on the right arm and use as little of the left as possible. In this case, the left arm is there to provide some stability; try not to pull with it.

◣ L-SHAPED PULL-UP

PRIMARY MUSCLES: Lats, core muscles, hip flexors **SECONDARY MUSCLES:** Upper back, biceps

STARTING POSITION: Grip the bar with your hands slightly wider than your shoulders. With your arms almost fully extended, stabilize your upper body. While keeping your knees straight, brace your core and lift your legs until they're parallel to the floor, creating an "L" shape with your body.

1: Using only your upper body, squeeze your shoulder blades together and pull yourself up until your chin is above the bar. Maintain the "L" shape throughout the movement.

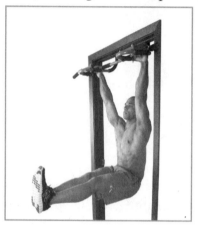

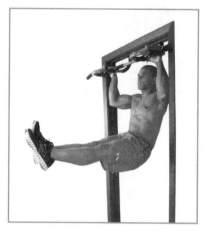

Slowly lower back to starting position while maintaining the leg position.

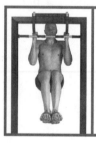

MODIFICATION: Bend your knees so that your thighs are parallel to the floor but your knees are bent 90 degrees.

◤ PULL-UP WITH LEG CURL

PRIMARY MUSCLES: Lats, biceps, abdominals   **SECONDARY MUSCLES:** Upper back, hip flexors

STARTING POSITION: Grip the bar with your hands slightly wider than your shoulders. Your arms should be close to fully extended and your knees bent and feet behind you.

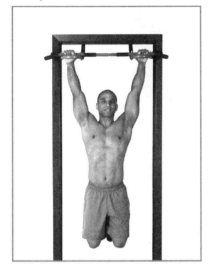

1: Initiate the movement by pinching your shoulder blades together and pulling up until your chin is above the bar. As you approach the top of your pull-up, curl your knees into your chest. Your knees should be curled in as high as you can comfortably get them.

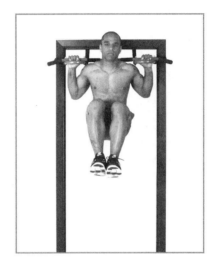

Lower your legs and then extend your arms to their starting position. Avoid swinging your legs during this portion.

PROGRESSION: Keep your legs straight and lift up to an "L" shape.

PROGRESSION: Pull up and lift your legs in one motion.

◨ HANGING BICEPS CURL

PRIMARY MUSCLES: Biceps **SECONDARY MUSCLES:** Lats, upper back
PREREQUISITE: Chin-Up, Isometric Hold

STARTING POSITION: Begin with a full chin-up (page 96) and hold at the top part of the movement.

1: Keep your shoulders stable and extend only at the elbow. Extend as much as you comfortably can.

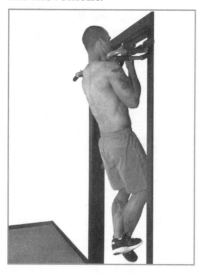

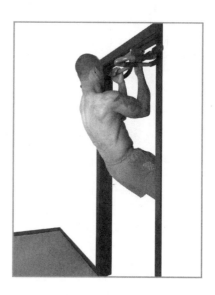

Curl back up to starting position by bending your elbows.

▰ ISOMETRIC HOLD (SIDE TO SIDE)

PRIMARY MUSCLES: Lats, upper back   **SECONDARY MUSCLES:** Biceps
PREREQUISITE: Pull-Up, Isometric Hold, Side-to-Side Pull-Up

STARTING POSITION: Begin at the top of a traditional pull-up. From here, lower your body so that the upper portion of both arms are parallel to the floor.

1: Bend one elbow while simultaneously extending the other, moving your body to one side. Your upper arms should still be parallel to the floor.

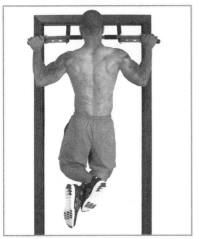

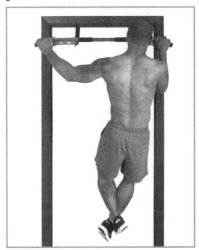

2: Reverse the movement all the way to the other side.

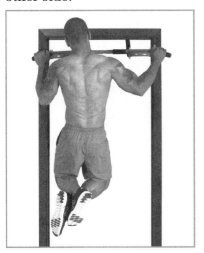

PULL-UP WITH PRESS-OUT

PRIMARY MUSCLES: Lats, upper back   **SECONDARY MUSCLES:** Biceps, deltoids
PREREQUISITE: Hanging Biceps Curl, Pull-Up, Isometric Hold

STARTING POSITION: Begin in the starting position for a pull-up.

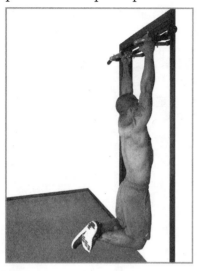

1: Squeeze your shoulder blades together and pull yourself up until your chin is above the bar.

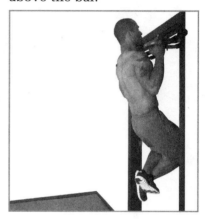

2: From the top position, extend your arms forward and push your body away from the bar as far as you comfortably can.

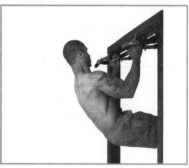

3: Pull yourself back in toward the bar.

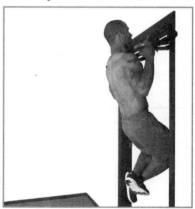

Lower back to starting position.

MODIFICATION: Try this with a chair pull-up.

PROGRESSION: Instead of lowering down, continue movements 2 and 3.

◣◢ PULL-UP WITH HIGH LEG RAISE

PRIMARY MUSCLES: Lats, upper back, rectus abdominis   **SECONDARY MUSCLES:** Biceps, hip flexors
PREREQUISITE: Pull-Up, Hanging Leg Curl

STARTING POSITION: Begin in a standard pull-up position.

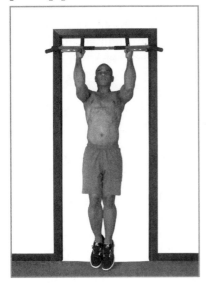

1: Initiate the movement by squeezing your shoulder blades together and lifting yourself up. As you pull yourself up, simultaneously swing your legs up until your feet are pointing toward the ceiling and your torso is parallel to the floor.

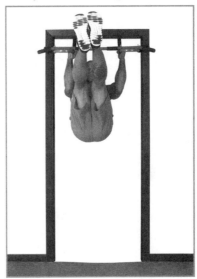

Lower your legs and return to starting position.

◣ SQUAT THRUST INTO PULL-UP

You can either jump enough to grab the bar, pause and pull-up, or you can jump and pull using the momentum from the jump to complete the pull-up.

PRIMARY MUSCLES: Lats, quads, upper back **SECONDARY MUSCLES:** Biceps, deltoids, chest
PREREQUISITE: Pull-Up, Jumping Pull-Up, Squat Thrust

STARTING POSITION: Stand upright facing the bar.

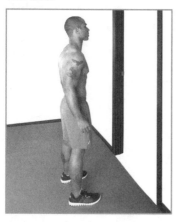

1–2: Begin a squat thrust by dropping to the floor and shooting your feet straight out.

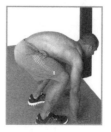 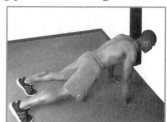

3: Pull your legs back in and jump.

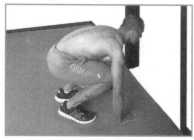

4–5: Catch yourself on the bar and complete the pull-up.

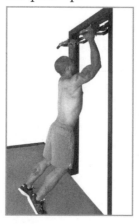 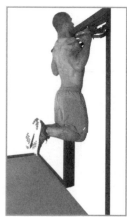

Drop right back into the next repetition.

PROGRESSION: Add a push-up to the bottom of the movement.

BUILDING UP TO PULL-UPS

If you're struggling with pull-ups, these exercises will help you build up to performing full pull-ups. These exercises can be performed with any hand position and can also be used as a substitute for the pull-up-based movements in your fitness program. They're listed progressively, from the easiest to the hardest, so be sure to work through each exercise in order to build toward the traditional pull-up.

SCAPULAR PULL-UP

PRIMARY MUSCLES: Rhomboids, upper back

STARTING POSITION: Grip the bar with your hands slightly wider than your shoulders. Your arms should be almost fully extended with your knees bent so that your feet are off the floor. From here, protract or release your shoulder blades as much as you can.

1: Making sure to avoid pulling with your arms for this movement, retract or squeeze your shoulder blades together.

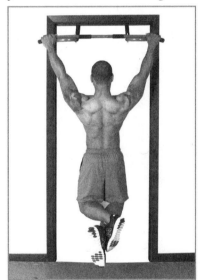

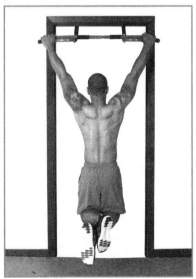

Slowly protract (release) the shoulder blades as much as you can.

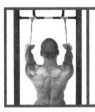 **MODIFICATION:** This exercise can be done with a rope/towel set-up (see page 114).

◨ ISOMETRIC HOLD

This exercise simply requires you to hold the top position of a pull-up for 5–10 seconds. The challenge here is getting to the top. Use one of the following methods: pull-up, partner-assisted pull-up, chair-assisted pull-up, jumping pull-up.

PRIMARY MUSCLES: Lats, biceps   **SECONDARY MUSCLES:** Upper back

THE POSITION: Assume the top pull-up position and hold. Your shoulder blades should be together and your chin should be over the bar.

MODIFICATION: Try the isometric hold at a quarter, a half or three-quarters of your full range of motion.

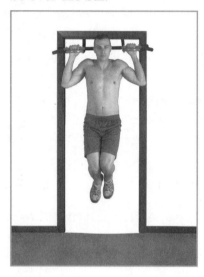

◣ PULL-UP WITH NEGATIVE FOCUS

Use one of the following methods to get to the top pull-up position: pull-up, partner-assisted pull-up, chair-assisted pull-up, jumping pull-up.

PRIMARY MUSCLES: Lats, upper back   **SECONDARY MUSCLES:** Biceps

STARTING POSITION: Assume the top pull-up position.

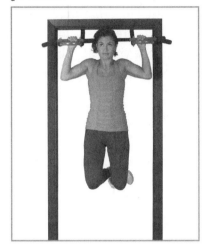

1–2: Over 5–10 seconds, slowly lower yourself. Make sure to keep your speed consistent throughout. Continue to lower until your arms are close to fully extended.

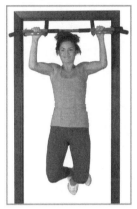 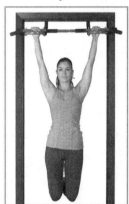

If performing more than one repetition at a time, use one of the methods discussed above to return to starting position.

PROGRESSION: Add a 2- or 3-second isometric hold at a quarter, a half and three-quarters of the way down. This will add 6–9 seconds to your total time.

◪ MODIFIED PULL-UP

This exercise (pictured with yoga straps) can be performed using anything from an old sweater to a pair of towels to yoga straps to jump ropes. Make sure that whatever you're using is long enough and strong enough to support your weight.

PRIMARY MUSCLES: Upper back, lats   **SECONDARY MUSCLES:** Biceps

STARTING POSITION: Hook up the straps to either side of the bar by pulling the end through one of the loops. Grip the end of each strap and wrap around your hand once to secure the grip. Fully extend your arms forward so that the rope is taut. Walk your legs forward until your feet are directly beneath the bar. At this point, there should be a straight line from your heels to your shoulders and the straps should be holding you up.

1: Initiate the movement by squeezing your shoulder blades together and pulling yourself up. Make sure that your body never gets completely vertical. The straps/pull-up bar should still be supporting your weight.

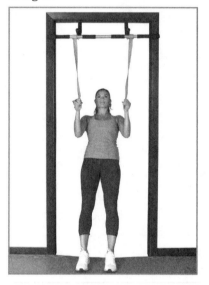

Extend your elbows and return to starting position.

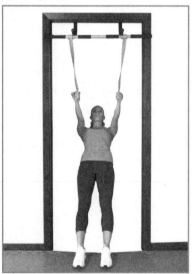

PROGRESSION: Start with your feet farther forward. The lower you are to the ground, the more difficult the movement will be.

◗◖ PARTNER-ASSISTED PULL-UP

PRIMARY MUSCLES: Lats, biceps   **SECONDARY MUSCLES:** Upper back

STARTING POSITION: Grip the bar with your hands slightly wider than your shoulders. Your arms should be almost fully extended. Have your partner stand behind you with their hands clasped together. Lift one leg and place it in your partner's hands, then lift the other leg and place it in your partner's hands as well. Your partner should assist you the entire way (if you're performing an isometric hold or a pull-up with negative focus, they should let go when you reach the top).

1: Initiate the movement by squeezing your shoulder blades together and pulling yourself up until your chest is within a few inches of the bar; your partner should still be holding your legs. Be sure to focus on your upper body and avoid pushing with your legs to generate lift.

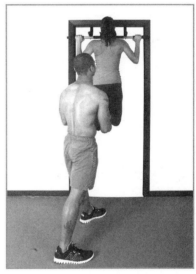

Slowly return to starting position. Try to rely on your partner as little as possible.

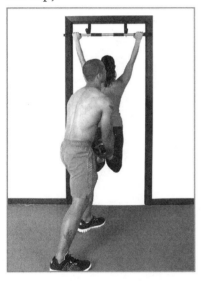

> **PROGRESSION:** Tell your partner to simply support your legs but provide no lift.

SHORT-RANGE PULL-UP (LOWER HALF)

Use this to build up to full-range-of-motion pull-ups. Try not to fall into the trap of turning this into your normal pull-up.

PRIMARY MUSCLES: Biceps, lats   **SECONDARY MUSCLES:** Upper back

STARTING POSITION: Grip the bar with your hands slightly wider than your shoulders. Your arms should be close to fully extended. Bend your knees in order to pick your feet up off the floor.

1: Initiate the movement by squeezing your shoulder blades together and pulling yourself up until each upper arm (from the shoulder to the elbow) is parallel to the floor, forming a "T" shape with your torso.

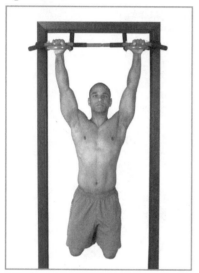

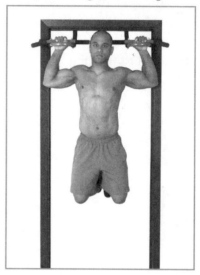

Extend down to starting position.

PROGRESSION: Pull yourself three-quarters of the way up.

SHORT-RANGE PULL-UP (UPPER HALF)

Use one of the following methods to get to the top pull-up position: pull-up, partner-assisted pull-up, chair-assisted pull-up, jumping pull-up.

PRIMARY MUSCLES: Biceps, lats   **SECONDARY MUSCLES:** Upper back

STARTING POSITION: Assume the top pull-up position.

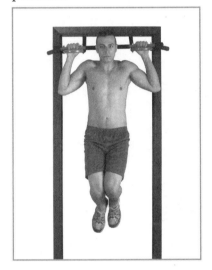

1: Lower yourself halfway down or until the upper part of each arm (from the shoulder to the elbow) is parallel to the floor, forming a "T" shape with your torso.

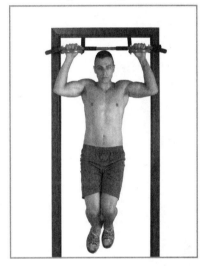

Pull back up to starting position.

> **PROGRESSION:** Lower yourself three-quarters of the way down.

CHAIR-ASSISTED PULL-UP

PRIMARY MUSCLES: Lats, biceps   **SECONDARY MUSCLES:** Upper back

STARTING POSITION: Place a chair slightly behind the pull-up bar. The chair should be high enough that you're close to the top position of a pull-up with your feet still on the chair. Begin by standing on the chair and securing yourself at the top of the bar. Shift onto your toes and lower yourself by extending your arms and bending your knees.

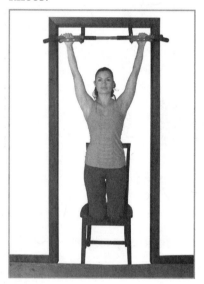

1: Squeeze your shoulder blades together and pull yourself up until your chin is above the bar. Keep your feet on the chair and push down onto the chair to provide any extra help if needed for the lift. Try to focus your energy on the upper body. Only use your legs as much as is necessary to complete the movement.

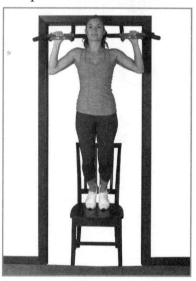

Bend your knees and lower yourself back down to starting position.

◣◢ BAND-ASSISTED PULL-UP

A stronger band will provide more assistance.

PRIMARY MUSCLES: Lats, biceps   **SECONDARY MUSCLES:** Upper back

STARTING POSITION: Place a chair behind the pull-up bar. Using a pair of exercise bands, hook the handles over the parallel bars. Step on the chair and grip the bar using the desired hand position. Stabilize your upper body near the top of the pull-up bar. Using one leg at a time, place your knees on the band and lower yourself by extending your arms.

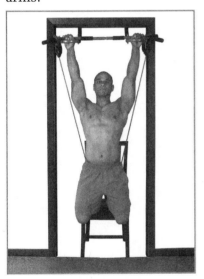

1: Initiate the movement by squeezing your shoulder blades together and pulling yourself up until your chin is above the bar.

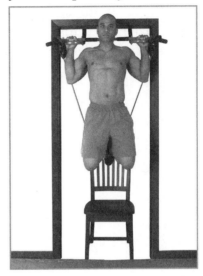

Lower back to starting position.

When you're finished with the exercise, pull up to the top and take one leg out at a time before placing them on the chair.

◣ JUMPING PULL-UP

This exercise can only be performed if you can stand under the bar with your arms fully extended and still not touch the bar. Also, this should only be attempted if the structure is secure. Some doorframes will be strong enough to handle your weight during a pull-up but not the added force resulting from the jump, so exercise caution.

PRIMARY MUSCLES: Lats   **SECONDARY MUSCLES:** biceps

STARTING POSITION: Stand under the bar with your arms extended. Your palms should be facing each other and in position to grab the parallel bars.

1: Keeping your arms extended, sit back into a squat and jump. The jump should be just enough to reach the bar.

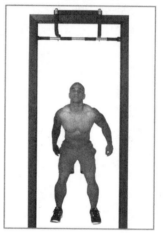

2: This part requires good timing: As your hands reach the level of the bar, simultaneously grab the bar and perform a standard pull-up.

Slowly lower yourself and drop softly back to the floor.

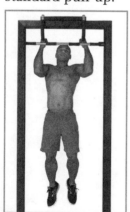 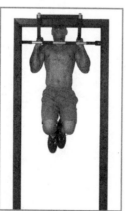

> **MODIFICATION:** Practice the movement by jumping and slapping the handles without gripping.

JUMPING PULL-UP (FEET ON FLOOR)

This exercise can only be performed if your feet are in contact with the floor while gripping the bar. A stable bench may be used.

STARTING POSITION: Stand directly underneath the bar. Extend your arms and grip the handles.

1: Bend your knees slightly and simultaneously jump and pull yourself up as high as you comfortably can.

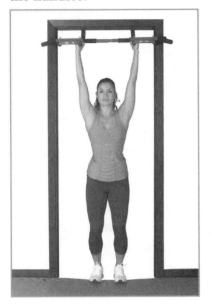

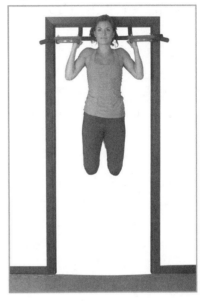

Control yourself back to starting position.

◤◥ HANGING ABDOMINAL EXERCISES

A pull-up bar can be great for working the abs and the entire core. This section will cover core exercises using the pull-up bar. As I covered earlier, there's a difference between exercises that are meant for the core (stabilizing the back and pelvis) and exercises specifically targeting the abdominals (curling movements). Exercises that require you to lift your legs with a straight back are designed for the core, and you need to focus on bracing your trunk. All of these exercises can be performed using hanging straps or by holding onto the bar.

TECHNIQUE

HANGING STRAPS: The hanging straps are a pair of straps that connect to the pull-up bar. Once connected, slip your arm into the strap so that the upper part of your arm (between the shoulder and the elbow) is resting comfortably in it and parallel to the floor.

HOLDING WITH THE ARMS: If you're holding yourself up, find a comfortable hand position (parallel is usually the easiest). With your arms almost fully extended, your back and legs should be straight and perpendicular to the floor. If your feet are touching the floor, you'll have to pull yourself up to a point where your feet are no longer on the floor. If you have a hard time holding yourself up but your feet are touching the floor, bend your knees in order to pick your feet up off the floor. Once you find a solid position, keep your upper body as stable as possible for the duration of the movement.

⬗ HANGING LEG CURL

PRIMARY MUSCLES: Abdominals, hip flexors

STARTING POSITION: Hang from the bar with both legs completely straight.

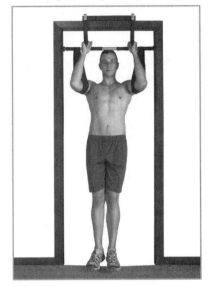

1: Keeping your upper body stable, squeeze your abdominal area and curl your knees into your chest as close as you can comfortably get them. Your upper body should be as stable as possible throughout the movement.

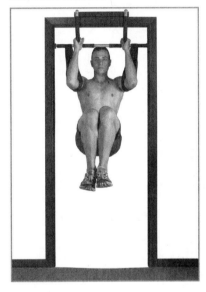

Slowly lower your legs.

MODIFICATION: Pull your legs up until your thighs are parallel to the floor.

◤ STRAIGHT-LEG RAISE

PRIMARY MUSCLES: Core, hip flexors

STARTING POSITION: Hang from the bar with your legs completely straight.

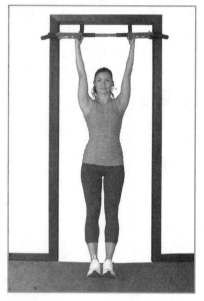

1: Brace your core and lift your legs up until they're parallel to the floor. Your body should be in an "L" shape with your knees completely straight. Pause for 1–2 seconds.

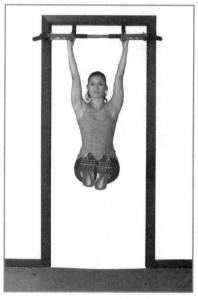

Slowly lower back to starting position.

> **MODIFICATION:** Bend your knees at the start. Make sure to maintain the same angle throughout the movement.
>
> **PROGRESSION:** Pause for 5 seconds when you reach the top.

◣ HANGING LEG CURL WITH ROTATION

PRIMARY MUSCLES: Abdominals, obliques   **SECONDARY MUSCLES:** Hip flexors

STARTING POSITION: Hang from the bar with your legs completely straight.

1: While curling your knees in toward your chest, rotate your torso in one direction. At the top of the movement, your torso should be rotated about 45 degrees with your knees as close to your chest as you can comfortably get.

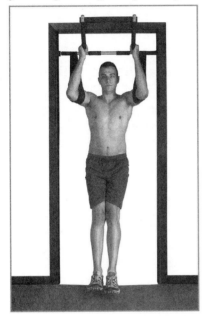

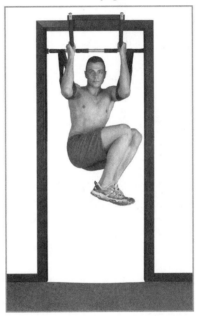

Slowly rotate back to starting position and lower your legs.

STRAIGHT-LEG RAISE SIDE TO SIDE

PRIMARY MUSCLES: Core   **SECONDARY MUSCLES:** Hip flexors

STARTING POSITION: Hang from the bar with your legs completely straight.

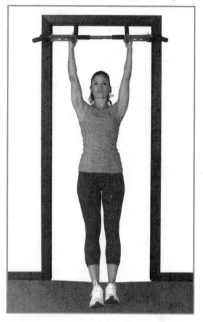

1: While keeping your knees straight, lift your legs up and across to one side. At the top of the movement, your legs should be slightly higher than parallel to the floor and your torso should be rotated 45 degrees. Try to lift and rotate at the same time.

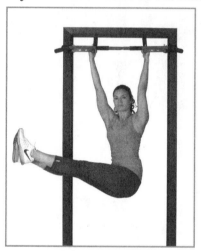

2: Slowly lower back to starting position and repeat to the other side.

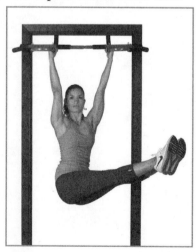

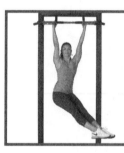

MODIFICATION: Shorten the range of motion on the leg raise.

ALTERNATE SINGLE-LEG RAISE

PRIMARY MUSCLES: Core, hip flexors

STARTING POSITION: Hang from the bar with your legs completely straight.

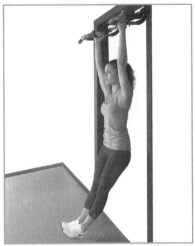

1: Lift one leg until it's parallel to the floor, keeping the other leg hanging down.

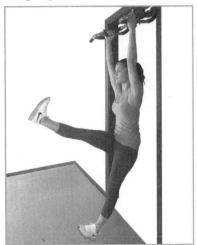

2: Slowly lower the leg and switch to the other side. Be sure to lower your leg all the way down before beginning the next repetition.

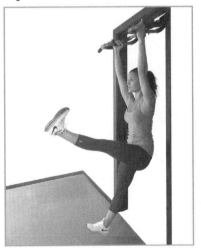

MODIFICATION: If flexibility is an issue, shorten the range of motion or bend your knee.

PROGRESSION: Make the movement more scissorslike and lift one leg as the other is lowering.

ALTERNATE SINGLE-LEG RAISE SIDE TO SIDE

PRIMARY MUSCLES: Core, obliques   **SECONDARY MUSCLES:** Hip flexors

STARTING POSITION: Hang from the bar with your legs completely straight.

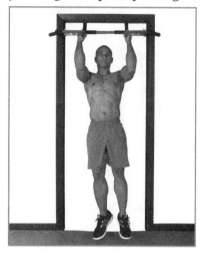

1: Lift one leg up and across your body. At the top of the movement, your leg should be higher than parallel to the floor. Pause at the top.

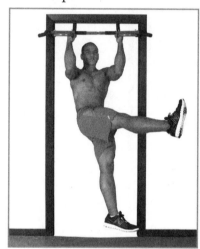

2: Slowly lower to starting position and lift your other leg.

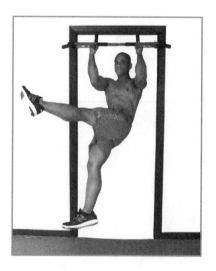

▰ OBLIQUE TWIST

This can be performed with or without hanging straps.

PRIMARY MUSCLES: Core

STARTING POSITION: Hang from the bar and raise your legs so that your thighs are parallel to the floor and your knees are bent 90 degrees.

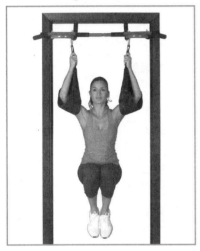

1: While maintaining the position of your legs, rotate your torso as much as you can.

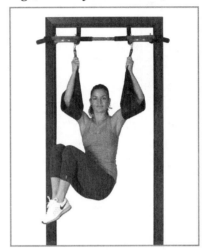

2: Twist all the way over to the other side without pausing in the middle.

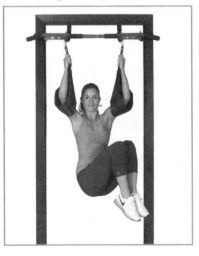

PROGRESSION: Straighten your legs so that your body is in an "L" shape.

◢◣ HALF CIRCLE

PRIMARY MUSCLES: Obliques, hip flexors

SECONDARY MUSCLES: Abdominals

STARTING POSITION: Hang from the bar with your legs straight.

1–2: While keeping your legs together and knees extended, swing your legs out to the side and draw as large of a half circle with your toes as you comfortably can. As your legs swing up, you should curl your trunk in a bit. At the top of the movement, your legs should be in line with your torso and your feet should be pointing up.

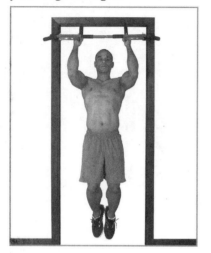

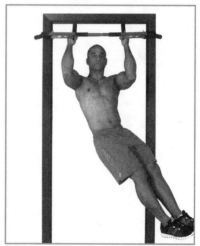

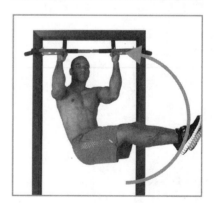

3: From the top position, lower your legs straight down and prepare to lift in the other direction.

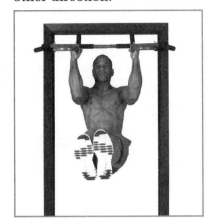

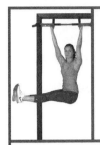

MODIFICATION: Don't curl your trunk. Brace your core and draw a half circle until your legs are parallel to the floor.

PROGRESSION: On the return, retrace the half circle to lower your legs.

◤ FULL CIRCLE

This can be performed with or without hanging straps.

PRIMARY MUSCLES: Obliques, hip flexors

SECONDARY MUSCLES: Abdominals

STARTING POSITION: Hang from the bar with your legs straight.

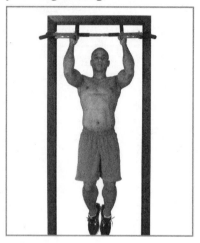

> **MODIFICATION:** Don't curl your trunk. Brace your core and draw a full circle with your legs.

1–2: While keeping your legs together and knees extended, swing your legs out to the side and draw as large of a circle with your toes as you comfortably can. As your legs swing up, you should curl your trunk a bit. At the top of the movement, your legs should be in line with your torso with your feet pointing up.

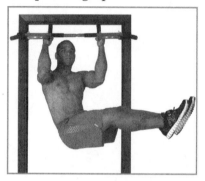

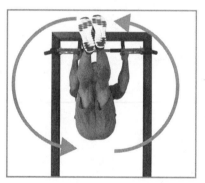

From the midpoint, continue drawing your circle by lowering your legs in the other direction. Each repetition should be one continuously smooth movement so try not to pause at the midpoint.

◪ LEG CURL WITH EXTENSION

This can be performed with or without hanging straps

PRIMARY MUSCLES: Abdominals, hip flexors

STARTING POSITION: Hang from the bar with both legs straight.

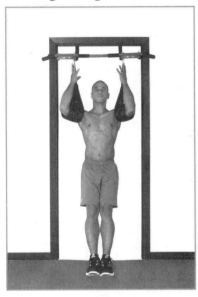

1: Keeping your upper body stable, squeeze your abdominal area and curl your knees into your chest.

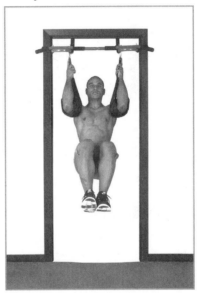

2: Keeping your abdominals curled, extend your knees so that your legs are completely straight and slightly higher than parallel to the floor.

Uncurl your trunk and slowly lower your legs.

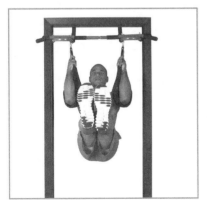

MODIFICATION: Don't curl your trunk at all.

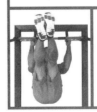

PROGRESSION: Curl your trunk enough so that your feet point up toward the ceiling

◧ HANGING OBLIQUE CRUNCH

PRIMARY MUSCLES: Obliques   **SECONDARY MUSCLES:** Abdominals

STARTING POSITION: Hang from the bar with both legs straight.

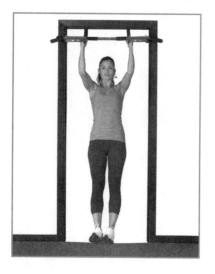

1: While keeping your upper body as stable as possible, squeeze your obliques on one side and lift your legs laterally to that side. Imagine that you're pulling your hip bone on one side up to the armpit on the same side.

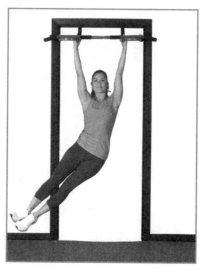

Slowly lower straight back down to starting position.

HANGING BICYCLE

PRIMARY MUSCLES: Abdominals **SECONDARY MUSCLES:** Hip flexors

STARTING POSITION: Grip the parallel bars and pull up until your elbows are bent 90 degrees. Curl your torso slightly and extend one leg so that it's parallel to the floor while pulling the opposite leg into your chest.

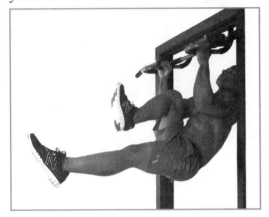

1: While maintaining the curl in your torso, simultaneously kick one leg straight out while pulling the other leg in.

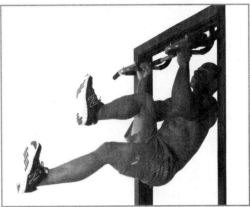

Repeat the motion, alternating your legs until you reach your desired repetitions or time. Maintain a consistent pace and try not to pause in between repetitions.

◣ HIGH TWIST

PRIMARY MUSCLES: Obliques   **SECONDARY MUSCLES:** Abdominals, upper back

STARTING POSITION: Grip the parallel bars and squeeze your shoulder blades together. Pull yourself up until your elbows are flexed about 90 degrees. From this point, swing your torso up so that it's parallel to the floor. Your hips and knees should be bent 90 degrees. Maintain this position throughout the exercise.

1: Twist your torso so that your knees lower to one side. Your torso should remain parallel to the floor while rotating as much as you comfortably can.

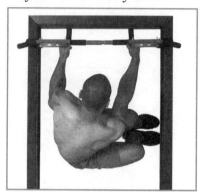

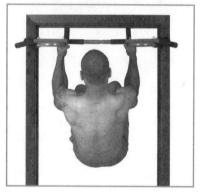

2: Rotate back to starting position and then over to the other side.

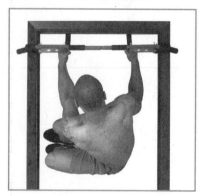

PROGRESSION: Instead of twisting, perform the bicycle movement.

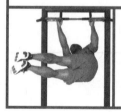

PROGRESSION: This can also be performed with straight legs.

◣ PUSH-UP-BASED EXERCISES

Push-ups are a great exercise for the chest, triceps and shoulders and complement pull-ups really well. Additionally, the need to stabilize your trunk makes push-ups an excellent core exercise. Like pull-ups, they're dynamic and can be progressed or modified to meet any person's needs. As is the case with the other sections, these exercises will get progressively more challenging. At the end of the section, I cover modifications if you're struggling with standard push-ups. If you have any shoulder or back pain when performing push-ups, I'd recommend getting it checked out by a physician or a specialist before continuing with the movement. If you're cleared to perform the exercise, you can try the modified push-ups found at the end of this section.

The doorframe pull-up bar is a terrific option for push-ups. When using one, place it on a flat surface. Grip the handles firmly and keep your wrists straight. More directions and variations can be found on page 169.

TECHNIQUE

HEAD POSITION: Keep your head in a neutral position. While moving, be sure to keep your head and neck in the same position and avoid extending your neck forward. Your eyes should be looking at the ground.

HAND POSITION: Changing your hand position will have an effect on how your muscles are being used. A close hand position will focus more on the triceps, while a very wide position will focus more on the chest. For the standard push-up, keep your hands right under your shoulders, perpendicular to the floor.

WRIST POSITION: For some people, push-ups are difficult because of the hyperextended wrist position. If you have limited range of motion or a previous injury, push-ups can be painful and cause unnecessary stress on the joint. If you fall into this category, you may try one of the following modifications:

1) Play with your hand position. Try a slightly wider or narrower position. Also, try rotating your hand. Slightly rotating internally or externally may alleviate stress.

2) Use the doorframe pull-up bar.

ELBOW POSITION: The direction that you move your elbows will also have an effect on the muscles being used. Unless otherwise noted, your elbows should both point and bend straight out to the side so that you're making a "T" shape with your arms and torso.

SHOULDER BLADE POSITION: As you lower into a push-up, retract (squeeze together) your shoulder blades.

LOWER BACK/TRUNK POSITION: It's important to brace your core throughout the movement. People commonly overarch their back, especially during the upward movement. Bracing will limit this.

FOOT POSITION: Foot position may vary, but make sure you're on your toes. A wider foot position will increase your base and make the exercise easier.

MOVEMENT

Once you're in position, initiate the movement by bending your elbows and lowering your chest to the floor. Be sure to maintain a neutral spine, as it's not uncommon for people to drop their hips and arch their back.

Inhale and lower your chest as far as is comfortable. Ideally, you should be able to lower to the point that your chest is about 3–4 inches off the floor, but make whatever adjustments you have to. It's more important that you work with a range that's comfortable for your shoulders.

On the way up, exhale as you push up through your palms while squeezing your chest. Make sure that you don't arch your back here, as it's a common error. Remember to brace your core.

◄► PUSH-UP

PRIMARY MUSCLES: Chest, triceps   **SECONDARY MUSCLES:** Shoulders, abdominals

STARTING POSITION: Place your hands on the floor directly under your shoulders and extend your legs behind you. Your hands and toes should be the only points of contact on the floor and your body should be in a neutral position, with a straight line from your shoulders, through your back and to your ankles.

1: Brace your core and bend your elbows to lower your chest until it's 3–4 inches off of the floor and your elbows are straight out to the sides.

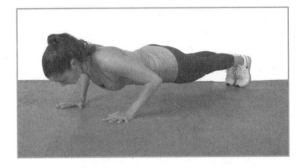

Push yourself up through your palms while squeezing your chest and returning to starting position.

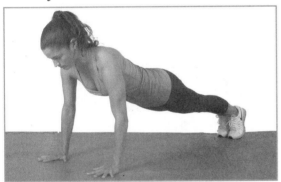

MODIFICATIONS: If you're struggling with standard push-ups, the following exercises are all great modifications. These can be used with all of the push-ups listed in the push-up series, not just the standard version.

- Perform the push-up with your knees on the floor.

- Perform the push-up from standing with your hands against a wall.

- Shorten the range you lower down, perhaps half to a quarter of the way down.

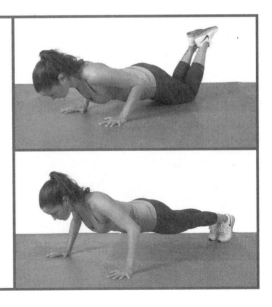

◣◥ WIDE PUSH-UP

A wider arm position will focus more on the chest and will have less triceps involvement.

PRIMARY MUSCLES: Chest   **SECONDARY MUSCLES:** Triceps, shoulders

STARTING POSITION: Begin in a prone (face-down) position with your hands and feet in contact with the floor. Your hands should be wider than your shoulders (6–12 inches wider than the standard push-up position).

1: Brace your core and initiate the movement by bending your elbows and lowering your chest to the floor. Your chest should be as close to the floor as you can comfortably get it.

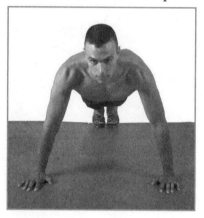

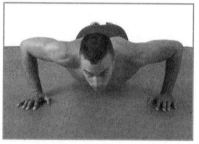

Press up through your palms and extend back to starting position.

PROGRESSION: When you reach the midpoint (don't touch the floor with your chest), stay in that position. From there, shift your body side to side by simultaneously bending one elbow while extending the other.

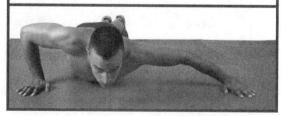

◤◢ DIAMOND PUSH-UP

PRIMARY MUSCLES: Triceps   **SECONDARY MUSCLES:** Shoulders

STARTING POSITION: Begin in a prone (face-down) position with your hands and feet being the only points of contact with the floor. Position your hands so that both index fingers and both thumbs are touching, forming a diamond shape.

1: Brace your core and bend your elbows, lowering your chest to 3–6 inches above your hands.

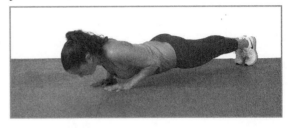

Squeeze your triceps and extend back up to starting position.

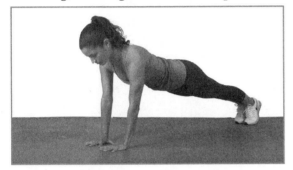

◤◢ TRICEPS PUSH-UP

PRIMARY MUSCLES: Triceps   **SECONDARY MUSCLES:** Chest, shoulders

STARTING POSITION: Begin in a prone (face-down) position with your hands and feet being the only points of contact with the floor. Unlike the previous exercises, your elbows should be pointing behind you for this exercise.

1: Brace your core and initiate the movement by bending your elbows and lowering your chest 2–3 inches from the floor. Your arms should stay close to your torso the entire time.

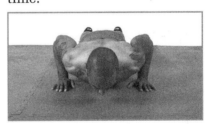

Push up through your palms back to starting position.

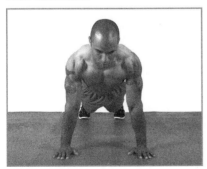

◣◥ STAGGERED PUSH-UP

This is a very flexible movement, so make any adjustments to the hand position to make it more comfortable.

PRIMARY MUSCLES: Chest   **SECONDARY MUSCLES:** Triceps, shoulders

STARTING POSITION: Begin in a prone (face-down) position with your hands and feet being the only points of contact with the floor. From this position, move one hand forward 3–6 inches. Move the other hand back 3–6 inches.

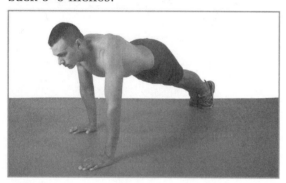

1: Brace your core and initiate the movement by bending your elbows and lowering your chest 3–6 inches off the ground. The lower arm will be closer to your body than your upper arm. You won't make a perfect "T" shape with your arms.

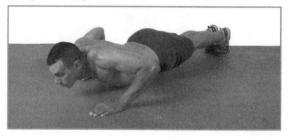

Squeeze your chest and drive up through your palms back to starting position. Perform all of your repetitions in one position and then switch over to the other position.

◀ POWER PUSH-UP

...s is an advanced exercise—exercise caution when attempting it. Please read all of the ...ections and follow them closely. Avoid if you have any joint injuries. It's important to ...d correctly. Begin by bending your elbows and bracing for the landing as you fall from ...top of the movement. When your hands touch the floor, your elbows should already be ...t and you should continue bending until you reach the bottom part of the movement. ...id landing with your arms straight. At the bottom of the movement, quickly explode ...k into the next repetition. The transition from landing to pushing back up should be ...ck. Try not to pause in between repetitions.

...IMARY MUSCLES: Chest   **SECONDARY MUSCLES:** Triceps, shoulders

...RTING POSITION: Begin in a standard ...sh-up position.

1: Brace your core and initiate the movement by bending your elbows and lowering your chest until it's 3–6 inches off the floor.

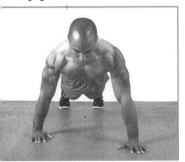

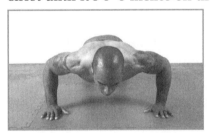

...While keeping your core engaged, drive ...through your palms as powerfully ...you can—your arms should be fully ...ended and your hands can be anywhere ...m 3–12 inches off of the floor.

MODIFICATION: Only push up 1–2 inches off the ground.

PROGRESSION: Begin with the same hand position as the Staggered Push-Up (page 142). For each repetition, switch the hand position in midair.

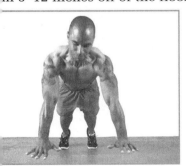

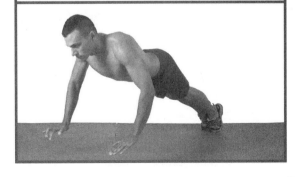

◣◢ PUSH-UP WITH ROTATION

PRIMARY MUSCLES: Chest, obliques   **SECONDARY MUSCLES:** Triceps, deltoids
PREREQUISITE: Push-Up, Plank with Rotation, Shoulder Touch

STARTING POSITION: Begin in a standard push-up position.

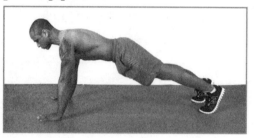

1: Bend your elbows and lower your chest to the floor.

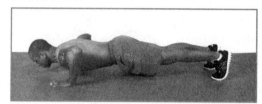

2–3: Press up through your palms and extend your elbows. As you approach the top of the push-up, lift one arm and swing it out to the side while rotating your entire body until you're facing the side with your feet staggered. The arm on the floor should be fully extended and your trunk should be straight and stable. Rotate back to starting position.

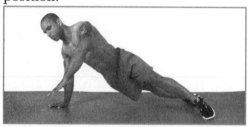

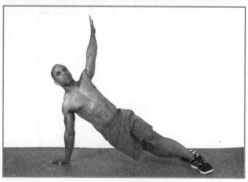

◣ TOTAL-BODY EXPLOSIVE PUSH-UP

PRIMARY MUSCLES: Chest   **SECONDARY MUSCLES:** Triceps, deltoids, quads, abs
PREREQUISITE: Power Push-Up, Plank

STARTING POSITION: Begin in a standard push-up position.

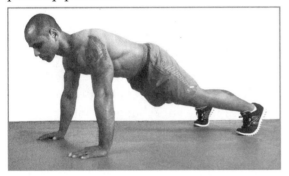

1: Bend your elbows and lower your chest to the floor. As you lower, bend your knees a bit as well.

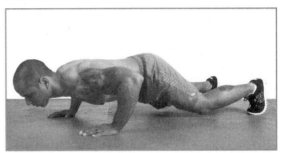

2: When you reach the bottom of the movement, explode up by driving up through your palms as well as extending your knees and pushing up from your legs until your hands and feet are as far off the ground as you can get them.

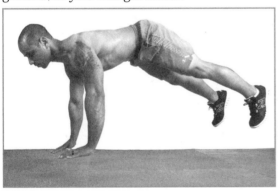

3: As you fall back to the floor, begin to bend your elbows and knees for a soft landing. Upon hitting the floor, you should be in the process of lowering into the next repetition.

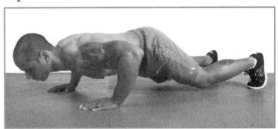

◼◼ LOWER-BODY EXERCISES

◼◼ SQUAT

PRIMARY MUSCLES: Quads, glutes   **SECONDARY MUSCLES:** Hamstrings, lower back

STARTING POSITION: Stand upright with your feet hip-width apart and your toes pointing straight ahead.

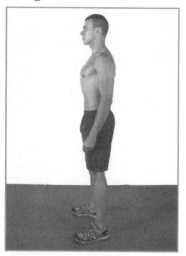

1: Brace your core and sit straight back, as if sitting in a chair, keeping your heels on the floor the entire time. Make sure that you're leaning forward as well; your torso should be bent forward at an angle from the hips, but make sure that your lower back is not overarched. Lower yourself until your thighs are close to parallel to the floor. Your heels should still be flat on the floor with your toes pointing straight ahead. Your knees should be in line with your toes but they shouldn't be in front of the toes.

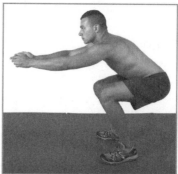

Engage your quads as well as your glutes and drive up through your heels back to starting position.

MODIFICATION: Begin with a wider stance and your toes pointed out slightly.

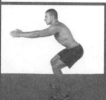 **MODIFICATION:** Go down half or three-quarters of the way.

◤◢ SPLIT SQUAT

The range of motion is variable for this exercise — go through a range that's comfortable for you. The distance between your legs will determine the balance of the muscles used. A narrower stance will focus more on the quads, while a wider stance will focus more on the glutes and hamstrings.

PRIMARY MUSCLES: Quads, glutes   **SECONDARY MUSCLES:** Hamstrings

STARTING POSITION: Stand upright with your feet about 6 inches apart. Split your legs apart by extending one leg behind the other. The front foot should be flat on the floor and you should be on your toes on the rear leg.

1: Initiate the movement by bending your rear leg and lowering straight down until your rear knee is as low as you can comfortably get it without touching the floor. Both knees should be bent at the same angle, but make sure that the front knee doesn't fall over the toes. Your torso should remain upright.

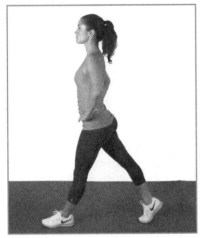

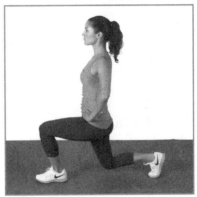

Drive up through your front heel and extend back up to starting position.

FORWARD LUNGE

PRIMARY MUSCLES: Quads, glutes **SECONDARY MUSCLES:** Hamstrings

STARTING POSITION: Stand upright with your feet about 6 inches apart.

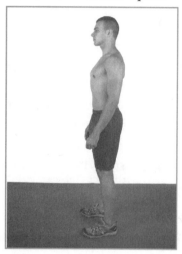

1: Step forward with one leg. As your lead foot hits the floor, raise the heel of your rear leg so that only your toes are touching the floor.

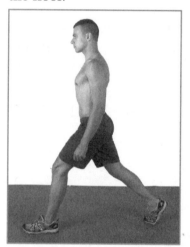

2: Initiate the movement by bending your rear knee and dropping straight down until your rear knee is as low as you can comfortably get it without touching the floor. Both knees should be bent at the same angle.

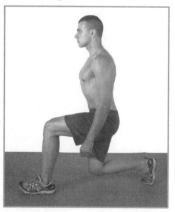

In one motion, drive up through the front heel back to starting position.

Once you're comfortable, try to combine movements 1 and 2 into one seamless motion.

◣◢ REVERSE LUNGE

PRIMARY MUSCLES: Quads, glutes   **SECONDARY MUSCLES:** Hamstrings

STARTING POSITION: Stand upright with your feet about 6 inches apart.

1: Take a step back with one leg, landing on your toes.

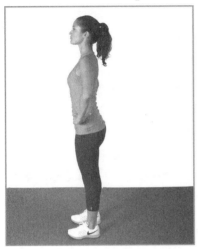

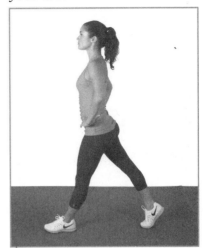

2: Initiate the movement by bending your rear knee and dropping straight down until your rear knee is as low as you can comfortably get it without touching the floor. Both knees should be bent at the same angle. Make sure that the back knee bends just as much as the front.

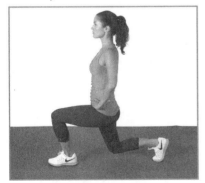

Drive up through the front heel and bring your rear leg back to starting position.

◣◢ BRIDGE

PRIMARY MUSCLES: Glutes   **SECONDARY MUSCLES:** Hamstrings, lower back

STARTING POSITION: Lie on your back on the floor with both knees bent and your feet on the floor but toes off the ground. Extend your arms along your sides.

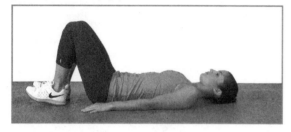

1: Brace your core, squeeze your glutes and lift your hips off the floor. Press your arms against the floor to assist with the movement. Your hips should be as high as you can comfortably get them without arching your back.

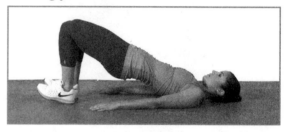

Lower back to starting position.

PROGRESSION: Keep your arms off the floor to decrease support.

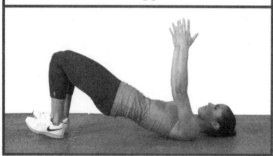

SINGLE-LEG BRIDGE

This has a shorter range of motion than the normal bridge (page 150).

PRIMARY MUSCLES: Glutes   **SECONDARY MUSCLES:** Lower back, hamstrings

STARTING POSITION: Lie on your back on the floor with both knees bent and your feet on the floor but toes off the ground. Lift one leg off the floor and pull it toward your chest with your arms. Hold it in place.

1: Brace your core and squeeze your glutes to lift your hips off the floor. Your hips should be as high as you can comfortably get them without arching your back.

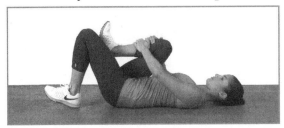

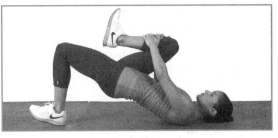

Slowly lower back to starting position.

◢◣ SINGLE-LEG SQUAT

PRIMARY MUSCLES: Quads, glutes   **SECONDARY MUSCLES:** Hamstrings, lower back

STARTING POSITION: While standing upright, lift one foot off the floor and bend your knee with your foot behind you.

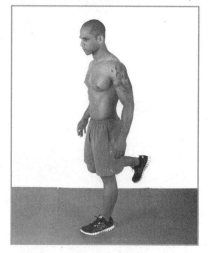

1: In one motion, sit back, lean forward and reach for the foot on the floor. Don't round your back, and make sure that your knees don't pass in front of your toes. Focus on the knee, the hip and the ankle while performing the movement.

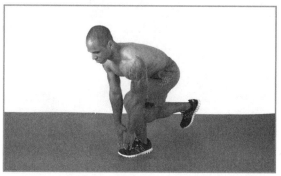

Maintaining your stability, drive back up through your heels to starting position. Do all of your repetitions on one leg before switching to the other leg.

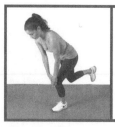

MODIFICATION: Instead of reaching for your foot, reach for the knee or shin of the standing leg.

◣ UPPER-BODY EXERCISES

◣ CHAIR DIP

PRIMARY MUSCLES: Triceps   **SECONDARY MUSCLES:** Shoulders

STARTING POSITION: Sit on the edge of a chair. Place your hands next to your body, grip the edge of the chair and walk your feet forward, lifting your bottom off the chair. Your torso should be straight and perpendicular to the floor while your legs should be straight with your heels on the floor. Point your elbows behind you.

1: Bend your elbows and lower your torso straight down. The height of the chair will determine how low you can go but, as a general rule, go as low as your shoulders will comfortably allow you to.

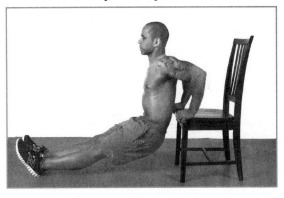

Squeeze your triceps and drive up through your palms back up to starting position.

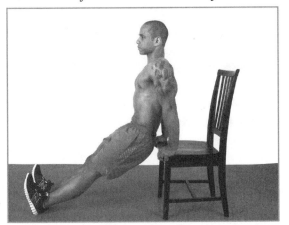

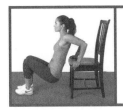

MODIFICATION: Bend your knees.

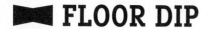 # FLOOR DIP

If you have any wrist issues, play with your hand position until you find one that's comfortable.

PRIMARY MUSCLES: Triceps   **SECONDARY MUSCLES:** Shoulders

STARTING POSITION: Sit on the floor with your knees bent. Your heels should be down and toes should be up off the floor. Place your hands on the floor behind your back with your elbows pointing back behind you, then lift your bottom off the floor.

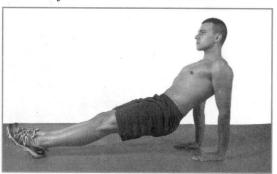

1: Bend your elbows and lower straight down until your bottom lightly touches the floor. Make sure that the movement happens at the elbow, not the shoulder.

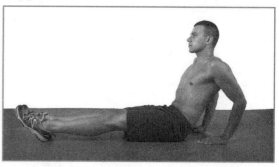

Squeeze your triceps and extend back up to starting position.

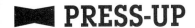 # PRESS-UP

PRIMARY MUSCLES: Triceps   **SECONDARY MUSCLES:** Abdominals

STARTING POSITION: Begin in a plank position, facedown with your forearms and toes on the floor. Your forearms should be flat on the floor with your hands open and palms down; your elbows should be bent 90 degrees with your upper arms perpendicular to the floor. There should be a straight line from your shoulders down to your ankles. Maintain a neutral spine.

1–2: Brace your core and press your palms into the floor while extending both elbows at the same time. Your elbows should be fully extended with your arms out in front of you. Make sure to maintain neutral spine for the entire movement.

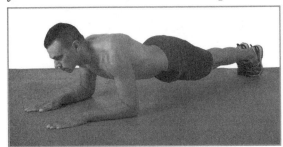

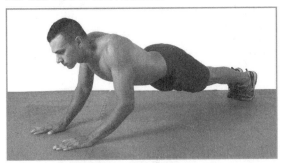

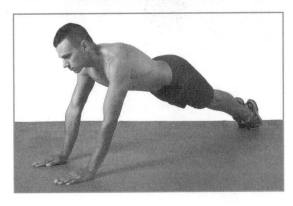

MODIFICATION: At the start of the movement, lower both knees to the floor.

MODIFICATION: Extend one arm at a time.

Bend your elbows and slowly lower back to starting position.

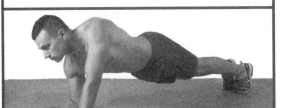

◥ PLANK WALK-UP

PRIMARY MUSCLES: Triceps, chest **SECONDARY MUSCLES:** Shoulders

STARTING POSITION: Begin in a plank position, facedown with your forearms and toes on the floor. Your forearms should be flat on the floor with your hands open and palms down; your elbows should be bent 90 degrees with your upper arms perpendicular to the ground. There should be a straight line from your shoulders down to your ankles. Maintain a neutral spine.

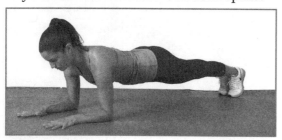

1: Lift one arm off the floor and place your hand directly under your shoulder. Extend your arm up and stabilize that arm and shoulder.

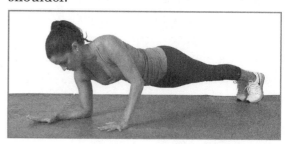

2: Lift the other arm and place that hand directly under your shoulder. Extend it as well until you're in a push-up position with your hands directly underneath your shoulders and your arms fully extended.

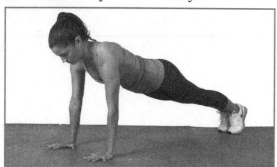

3: Begin the descent by bending whichever arm you started with and lowering it until the forearm is flat on the floor. Try to remain as stable as possible. Fight the urge to rotate or shift your weight more than is absolutely necessary.

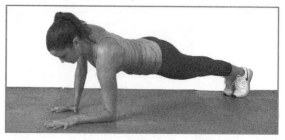

Lower the other arm until you're back in starting position. Be sure to alternate your lead arm so that your arms get equal work.

PROGRESSION: Add a push-up every time you reach the top of the movement.

STANDING WALK-OUT

PRIMARY MUSCLES: Chest, triceps **SECONDARY MUSCLES:** Abdominals

STARTING POSITION: Stand upright with your feet shoulder-width apart.

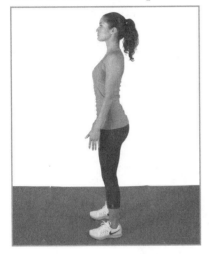

1–2: Bend down and place your palms on the floor as close to your feet as you can. From here, walk your arms forward until you're facedown with a straight line from your shoulders to your ankles. Your arms should be fully extended and directly under your shoulders.

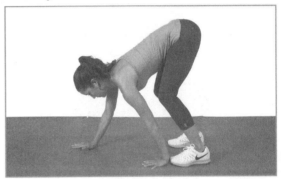

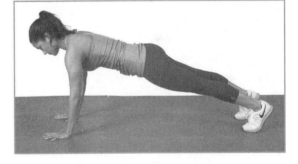

Walk your hands all the way back so they're in front of your feet and extend back up to starting position.

PROGRESSION: Walk your hands forward as much as you comfortably can before walking them back to your feet.

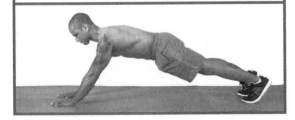

⋈ HANDSTAND SHOULDER PRESS

PRIMARY MUSCLES: Deltoids   **SECONDARY MUSCLES:** Triceps
PREREQUISITE: Pike Press, Push-Up

STARTING POSITION: While facing a wall, place your hands on the floor about 6 inches away from the wall. Kick your legs up so that you're upside down with your heels touching the wall behind you. Keep your legs straight and your arms fully extended.

1: Bend your elbows and slowly lower yourself as much as is comfortable.

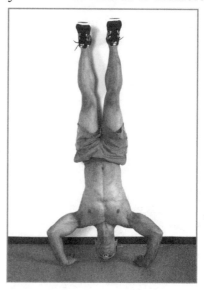

Press back up to starting position.

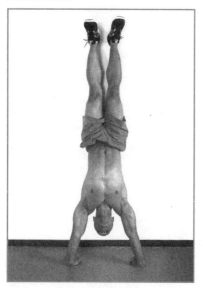

◤◢ PLANK-BASED EXERCISES

The plank is one of the most useful and effective core exercises. As mentioned earlier in the book, core exercises are those that focus on the stabilization of the trunk and pelvis. Planks accomplish this by engaging your core muscles in order to fight the forces of gravity to maintain a neutral spine.

Bracing the abdominals is necessary whenever you're performing a core exercise. Bracing involves contracting all of the muscles in the abdominal wall in order to stabilize the trunk. To do this, imagine that you're bracing for the impact from a punch. You want to tighten all of your trunk muscles and hold. Maintain this contraction throughout the entire plank.

TECHNIQUE

HEAD AND NECK POSITION: Your head should be in a neutral position facing the floor.

SHOULDER POSITION: Your shoulder blades should be held together throughout the exercise.

ARM POSITION: For a typical plank, your forearms are flat on the floor and parallel to each other. Elbows should be bent 90 degrees with your upper arms perpendicular to the floor.

TRUNK AND LOWER BACK POSITION: You should maintain a neutral position with your trunk and lower back throughout the exercise, whether it's static or dynamic. Your torso should be parallel to the floor.

LEG POSITION: Your legs should be fully extended with your toes on the floor.

MOVEMENT

The plank is a static or isometric exercise, meaning that once you're in position, you're not actively moving. Instead of moving, your muscles are fighting the forces of gravity or some form of external resistance in order to maintain a position. Keep your torso as close to parallel to the floor as you can. Imagine that you're trying to balance a pot of coffee on your back. A plank is typically held for anywhere from 5–60 seconds.

BREATHING

Since there's no active movement, try to maintain a consistent breathing pattern throughout the exercise. Inhale for 1–2 seconds and exhale for 1–2 seconds.

COMMON PROBLEMS

PROBLEM: The purpose of the plank is to maintain a stable spine with the torso parallel to the ground. It's not uncommon for a person to either lift the hips too high or to arch the back and lower the hips to the floor. Each one positions the body in a way that makes holding the position easier, but you lose many of the benefits.

SOLUTION: If you're having a problem with the position, try holding the plank with one or both knees on the floor. In this case, begin in a normal plank position and then lower your knee(s) to the floor.

PROBLEM: You're experiencing lower back pain.

SOLUTION: This may or may not be a sign of something more serious. I'd recommend getting your back looked at by a doctor before moving forward. If you're cleared to exercise but experience pain in the lower back, there are a couple of steps you can take. First, retry the plank but focus again on bracing your core. Second, determine when the pain starts. If it begins immediately, then you should modify the movement by dropping your knees to the floor. If the pain happens after a certain amount of time (10 seconds, for example), then hold the plank for that amount of time and work toward increasing the length of time that you can hold a plank pain-free.

PROBLEM: Shaking. It's not uncommon for your body to begin involuntarily shaking when trying a new exercise. There's nothing wrong with this—it's simply your body trying to figure out what to do. The shaking should stop once you're more comfortable with the exercise.

PROBLEM: You're experiencing shoulder pain.

SOLUTION: First, make sure that you squeeze your shoulder blades together and that your arms are in the correct position. If you're still experiencing pain, you can try the plank with your arms fully extended. In this case, your hands should be directly under your shoulders and your elbows should be extended.

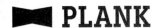 # PLANK

PRIMARY MUSCLES: Core   **SECONDARY MUSCLES:** Lower back

THE POSITION: Lie facedown on the floor. Place your forearms flat on the floor with your upper arms close to your torso. Your feet should be dorsiflexed with your toes on the floor. Brace your core and lift your body off the floor; only your forearms and toes should be in contact with the floor. Make sure to maintain neutral position throughout your body with your torso parallel to the floor. Your elbows should be bent 90 degrees with your upper arms perpendicular to the floor. Hold this position for the duration of the exercise.

MODIFICATION: Lower your knees to the floor.

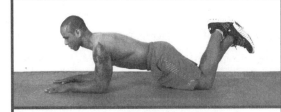

PROGRESSION: Extend your arms forward while keeping your torso parallel to the floor.

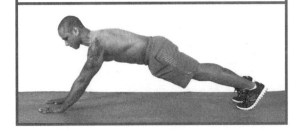

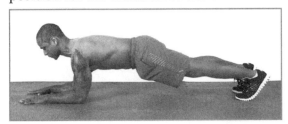

PLANK WITH ARM EXTENSION

PRIMARY MUSCLES: Core **SECONDARY MUSCLES:** Shoulders, lower back

STARTING POSITION: Lie facedown on the floor. Place your forearms flat on the floor with your upper arms close to your torso. Your feet should be dorsiflexed with your toes on the floor. Brace your core and lift your body off the floor; only your forearms and toes should be in contact with the floor.

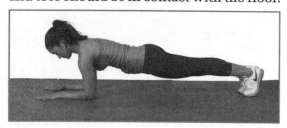

1: Staying as stable as you can, lift one arm off the floor and extend it forward. Keep your body level and your torso parallel to the floor. Pause for 1–2 seconds. Fight the urge to shift your weight or to rotate.

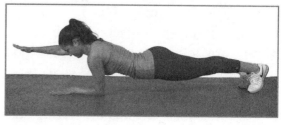

Lower the arm back to starting position and lift the other arm.

SIDE PLANK

This can be performed as a static (isometric) exercise or for repetitions.

PRIMARY MUSCLES: Obliques, abdominals   **SECONDARY MUSCLES:** Lower back

THE POSITION: Lie on your side with your forearm on the floor. Your forearm should be perpendicular to your body. Hips should be touching the floor and your legs should be straight with your feet stacked on top of each other. Brace your core and lift your hips off the floor. Your back should be straight and the only points of contact with the floor should be your feet and your forearm. Keep your top arm at your side.

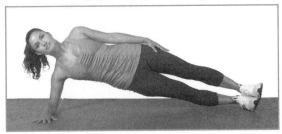

Lower back to starting position. Lightly touch your hip to the floor.

MODIFICATION: Place the top arm on the floor in front of you to add support.

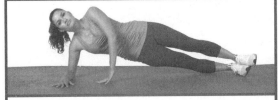

MODIFICATION: Bend the bottom knee behind you and keep the knee on the floor.

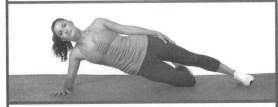

PROGRESSION: Lift your top leg off the bottom leg.

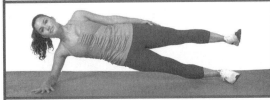

PROGRESSION: Externally rotate the bottom arm so that your forearm is in line with your body.

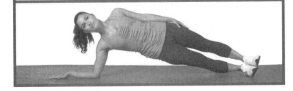

PLANK TO SIDE PLANK

PRIMARY MUSCLES: Core   **SECONDARY MUSCLES:** Lower back, shoulders

STARTING POSITION: Assume a plank position on your hands. Make sure your feet are about 8–12 inches apart.

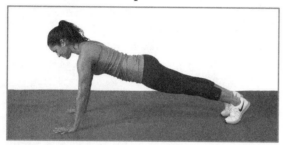

1–2: Lift one arm off the floor and rotate into a side plank position, raising your top arm to the ceiling.. Both feet should fall flat to the side and staggered next to each other. At the top of the movement, your back should be straight and the bottom arm should be perpendicular to your body.

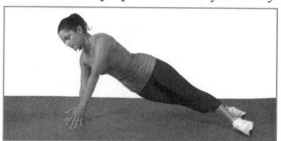

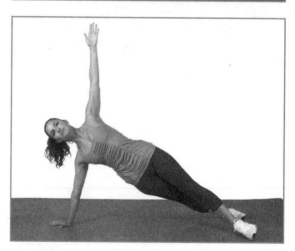

Rotate back to starting position and repeat on the other side.

MODIFICATION: Drop your knees to the floor.

PROGRESSION: Add 2–5 side plank repetitions every time you rotate.

ABDOMINAL EXERCISES

CRUNCH

PRIMARY MUSCLES: Abdominals   **SECONDARY MUSCLES:** Obliques

STARTING POSITION: Lie on your back with your knees bent and your feet on the floor. Place your hands together behind your neck or across the front of your neck, under your chin.

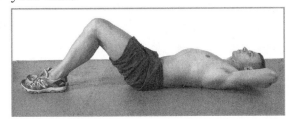

1: Curl your trunk so that you bring your rib cage to your pelvis. At the top of the movement, you should be curled at the trunk and your shoulders should be 3–4 inches off the floor. Make sure to keep your head and neck in a neutral position throughout the exercise, and fight the urge to push your neck forward.

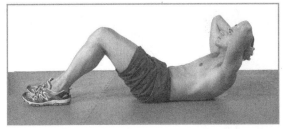

Extend back to starting position.

BICYCLE CRUNCH

PRIMARY MUSCLES: Abdominals, obliques   **SECONDARY MUSCLES:** Hip flexors

STARTING POSITION: Lie on your back with your arms interlocked behind your head. One leg should be fully extended but lifted off the floor; the other leg should be bent and in toward your chest. Rotate your torso so that your knee is touching the opposite elbow.

1: Simultaneously kick out the knee that's in and pull in the leg that's extended while also rotating your upper body, touching elbow to knee.

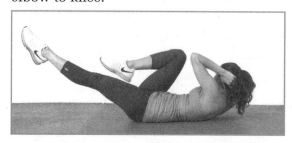

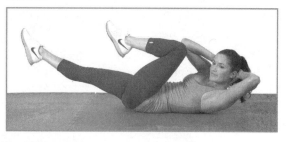

Once you begin the movement, keep alternating until you reach the desired number of repetitions.

> **MODIFICATION:** Shorten the leg extension.

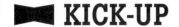 # KICK-UP

PRIMARY MUSCLES: Abdominals   **SECONDARY MUSCLES:** Lower back

STARTING POSITION: Lie on your back with your legs fully extended and your feet pointing up toward the ceiling. Your arms should be flat on the floor along your sides.

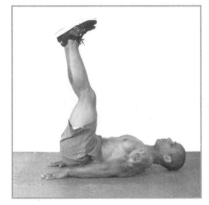

1: Initiate the movement by pressing your arms into the floor while lifting your hips off the floor. Your hips should be as high as you can comfortably raise them while keeping your feet pointing straight up toward the ceiling.

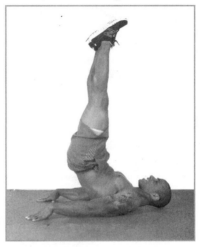

Slowly lower your hips back to starting position.

MODIFICATION: Bend your knees.

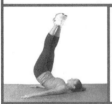 **PROGRESSION:** Add a rotation to the top of the movement.

◗◖ LEG CURL

PRIMARY MUSCLES: Abdominals   **SECONDARY MUSCLES:** Hip flexors, lower back

STARTING POSITION: Lie on your back with your legs fully extended and elevated 6–12 inches off the floor. Your arms should be flat on the floor by your sides.

1: Curl your knees into your chest and lift your hips off the floor. Your hips and knees should be bent as much as you comfortably can.

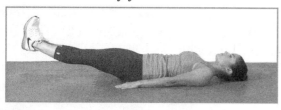

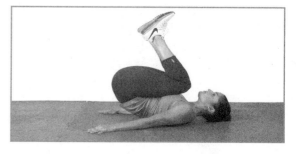

MODIFICATION: Shorten the range of motion.

PROGRESSION: Add a kick-up to the top of the movement.

Lower your hips and extend your legs back to starting position.

◗◖ TOTAL-BODY CRUNCH

PRIMARY MUSCLES: Abdominals, obliques   **SECONDARY MUSCLES:** Hip flexors

STARTING POSITION: Lie on your back with your arms fully extended behind you and your legs extended.

1: Swing your arms forward and crunch up while simultaneously curling your knees in. At the top of the movement, your knees should be curled into your chest while your torso should be curled up with your shoulders 3–6 inches off the floor.

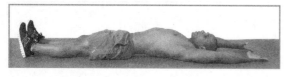

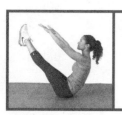

PROGRESSION: Sit up and make a "V" shape.

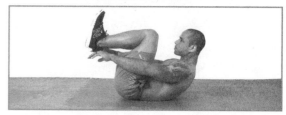

Simultaneously extend both your arms and legs back to starting position.

DOORFRAME PULL-UP BAR FLOOR EXERCISES

PUSH-UP WITH BAR

PRIMARY MUSCLES: Chest   **SECONDARY MUSCLES:** Triceps, shoulders

STARTING POSITION: Assume a facedown position with your hands gripping the wide ends of the bar. Your torso should be in a neutral position and your legs should be extended behind you.

1: Brace your core and bend your elbows out to the side, lowering your chest as much as you can while maintaining a stable position.

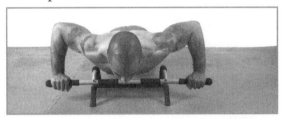

Drive up through your palms back to starting position.

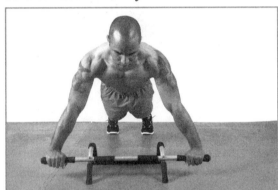

MODIFICATION: Place your knees on the floor.

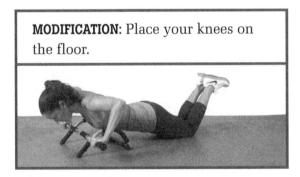

◤ DIP WITH BAR

PRIMARY MUSCLES: Triceps **SECONDARY MUSCLES:** Shoulders

STARTING POSITION: Sit down in front of the parallel bars. Grip the parallel bars with your hands and place your feet on the floor. Lift yourself up so that your feet are on the floor, your bottom is off the floor and your arms are fully extended along your sides.

1: Keeping your back perpendicular to the floor, bend your elbows straight back and lower yourself as much as you comfortably can without touching the floor.

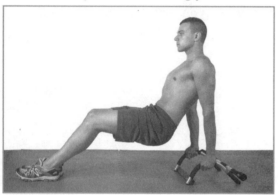

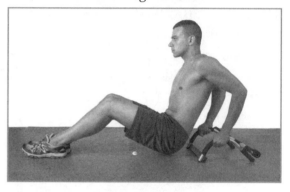

Press up through your palms and extend back up to starting position.

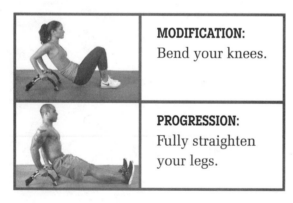

MODIFICATION: Bend your knees.

PROGRESSION: Fully straighten your legs.

◤ PRESS-UP WITH BAR

PRIMARY MUSCLES: Triceps **SECONDARY MUSCLES:** Core muscles

STARTING POSITION: Assume a facedown position and grip the bar with your hands about shoulder-width apart. Grip the bar with your palms facedown and turn your elbows in so that they face your toes. Your torso should be in a neutral position with your legs extended and toes on the floor as if for a push-up.

1: Keeping your elbows facing your body, brace your core and lower yourself by bending your elbows. Your elbows should bend 90 degrees or more. Maintain a neutral trunk position throughout. Don't allow your elbows to flare out to the sides. The entire movement consists of bending and extending your elbows, so avoid any other movements.

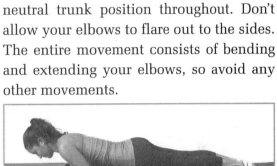

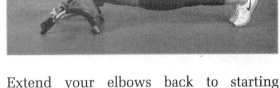

Extend your elbows back to starting position.

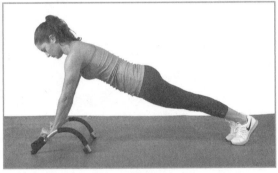

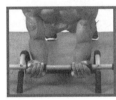

PROGRESSION: Try this with your palms facing you.

CORE WALK-OUT

PRIMARY MUSCLES: Core

STARTING POSITION: Assume a facedown position and grip the bar with your hands about shoulder-width apart. Your arms should be fully extended with your hands directly under your shoulders; your torso should be in a neutral position with your legs extended and toes on the floor. Brace your core.

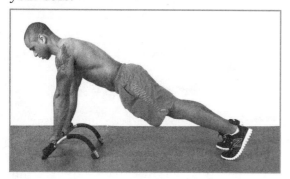

1–2: While maintaining a neutral and stable trunk, walk your feet backward. Keep your elbows locked in position so that the movement comes from your shoulders. Walk back as far as you comfortably can while maintaining a stable trunk.

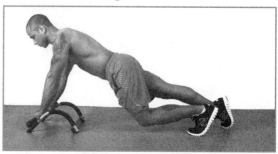

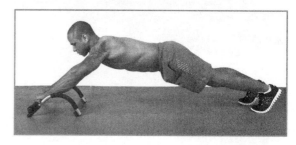

Slowly walk your feet back to starting position.

FRAME-ASSISTED SIT-UP

PRIMARY MUSCLES: Abdominals, hip flexors **SECONDARY MUSCLES:** Obliques

STARTING POSITION: Secure your feet in the bottom of the device by placing your feet below the bar. While keeping your heels on the floor, lift your toes so that the top of your feet touch the bar. This should secure you in place.. Lie on your back with arms behind your head.

1: Engage your abdominal muscles and sit up until your torso is 70–80 degrees. Your back should be straight.

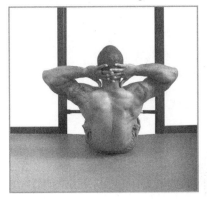

Slowly control back to starting position.

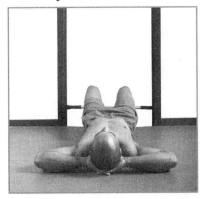

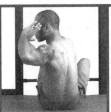

PROGRESSION: Add a twist at the top of the moment.

PROGRESSION: Stand at the top of the movement. Your feet will naturally release themselves from the bar.

▰ CALF RAISE

PRIMARY MUSCLES: Calves

STARTING POSITION: Stand with the balls of your feet on the bar. Lightly touch a wall or chair for balance. Take one foot off the bar and flex the ankle of the standing foot so that your heel is below the level of the bar.

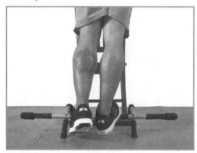

1: Squeezing your calf, extend your ankle and raise your heel as high as you can. Keep your leg straight throughout the movement.

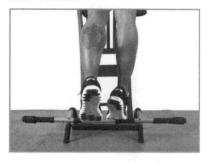

Lower back to the starting position.

> **MODIFICATION:** Perform both legs at the same time.

▰ LEG EXTENSION

PRIMARY MUSCLES: Quads   **SECONDARY MUSCLES:** Core

STARTING POSITION: Assume a facedown position with your hands on the floor and toes on the bar. Your legs should be fully extended and your arms should be extended with your hands under your shoulders.

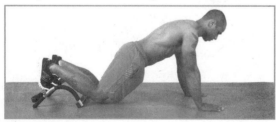

1: Bend your knees while keeping your torso parallel to the floor. Lower until your knees are 2–3 inches off of the floor.

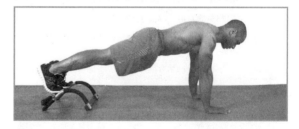

Squeeze your quads and extend back to starting position.

ALTERNATE-GRIP PUSH-UP WITH BAR

PRIMARY MUSCLES: Chest, triceps   **SECONDARY MUSCLES:** Shoulders

STARTING POSITION: Grip the wide end of the bar with one hand and grip the parallel bar with the other. Your body should be facedown with your torso in a neutral position, your legs extended behind you and your toes on the floor.

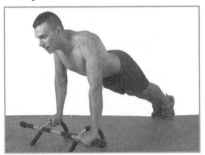

1: Bend both elbows and lower your chest as far as you comfortably can. As you lower, your wide arm should be bent out to the side while your parallel arm should be close to your body.

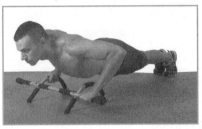

Extend back up to starting position and switch hand positions.

PIKE PRESS

PRIMARY MUSCLES: Shoulders   **SECONDARY MUSCLES:** Triceps

STARTING POSITION: Grip the parallel bars in a facedown position with your toes on the floor. Walk your feet forward, lifting your hips up. Try to keep your legs as straight as you can. Your body should create an inverted "V" with the bend at your hips. Your arms should be fully extended.

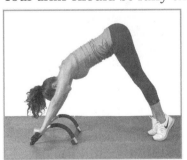

1: Bend your elbows and lower your head until it's in line with your hands. Pivot on your toes and try to maintain your back position as well as your straight legs.

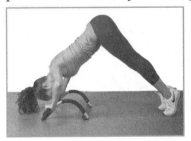

Press through your palms and extend your elbows until you reach starting position.

◣◗ CARDIO-CONDITIONING EXERCISES

The exercises in this section are all ideal for adding to a cardio-conditioning program. The purpose of these conditioning exercises is to increase your heart rate quickly and efficiently. These can be added to interval training as well as circuit-training programs. These are all athletic movements that require varying degrees of skill. Exercise caution and, if you have any joint pain or injuries, please consult your doctor before proceeding.

Each exercise in this section lists prerequisite exercises that you should be comfortable with prior to attempting these.

◣◗ SPEED SQUAT

PREREQUISITE: Squat

STARTING POSITION: Stand upright with your feet hip-width apart. Your toes should be pointing straight ahead and your elbows should be bent 90 degrees. Keep these angles throughout the exercise.

1: While keeping your elbows bent, swing your arms down. Using the momentum generated by the arm swing, sit back into a three-quarter squat. You should be on your heels.

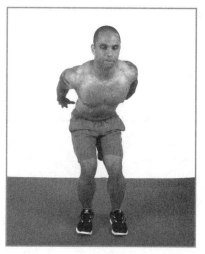

2: As soon as you reach the bottom of the movement, without pausing, quickly transition by swinging your arms back up. Using the momentum generated by your arms, extend your legs until you're on your toes.

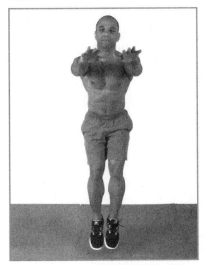

> **PROGRESSION:** Jump using the same technique. These jumps should be shorter and quicker.

3: As soon as you reach the top, without pausing, quickly transition back down by swinging your arms again.

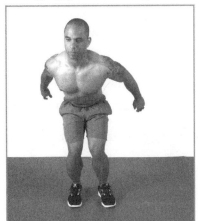

◤ SKATER

PREREQUISITE: Single-Leg Squat, Forward Lunge

STARTING POSITION: Stand with your feet about hip-width apart and sit back into a half squat.

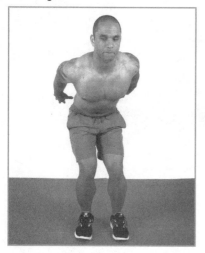

1: Lift your right leg off of the floor and drive off your left leg laterally into a small hop. Land on your right leg. The landing should be soft, with your knee bent and in position to jump again. Your left leg should not touch the floor.

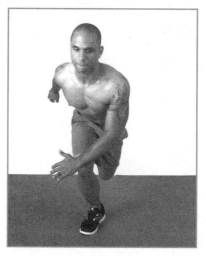

2: As soon as you land, drive off the right leg laterally back to the left side.

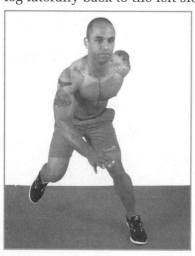

MODIFICATION: Land on both legs each time.

PROGRESSION: Increase the lateral distance.

SHOULDER TOUCH

PREREQUISITE: Push-Up, Plank with Arm Extension

STARTING POSITION: Begin in a push-up position. Keep your torso neutral and brace your core.

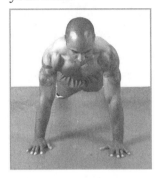

1: Keeping your body as stable as possible, lift one arm and touch the opposite shoulder. Fight the urge to shift your weight or to rotate.

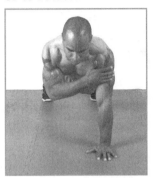

Lower your arm back to starting position and quickly lift the other arm.

MOUNTAIN CLIMBER

PREREQUISITE: Plank, Push-Up, Split Squat

STARTING POSITION: Begin facedown with your hands on the floor underneath your shoulders; your arms should be fully extended. One leg should be fully extended with the toes on the floor. The other leg should be in near your chest, bent at the knee and hip, also on your toes.

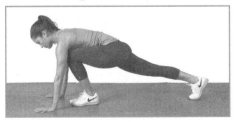

1: Simultaneously kick one leg straight back while pulling the other leg into your chest. Keep your torso stable and parallel to the floor throughout the movement.

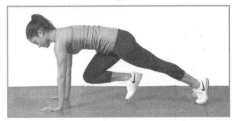

Continuously repeat the movement until you reach the desired time or repetition count.

◣ HIGH KNEES

PREREQUISITE: Mountain Climber, Speed Squat

STARTING POSITION: Stand upright and bend your elbows 90 degrees.

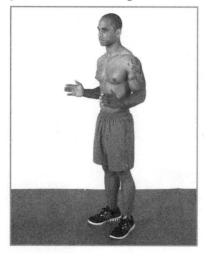

1–2: Begin running in place. As you run, pick your knees up so that your thighs are parallel to the floor. At the same time, make sure that your arms are swinging straight forward and back from your shoulders. Your arms and legs should be in sync so when you lift your right leg, your left arm should be swinging up as well.

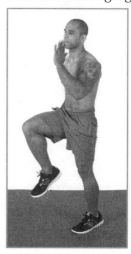 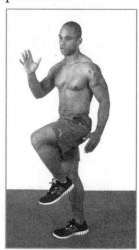

MODIFICATION: Take shorter steps.

◤◥ SQUAT JUMP

PREREQUISITE: Squat, Speed Squat

STARTING POSITION: Stand upright with your feet hip-width apart and your toes pointing straight ahead.

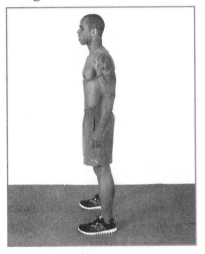

1: Swing your arms down while simultaneously sitting back into a squat.

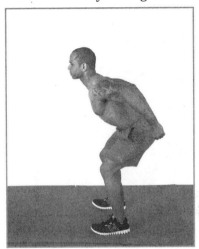

2: Once you reach the bottom of the squat, swing your arms back up while driving up through your heels and exploding into a jump. At the top of your jump, your legs should be fully extended.

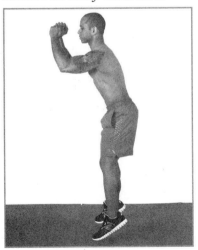

As you begin your descent, swing your arms down and begin to bend your knees. You should land softly and quietly in a squat position, with your knees and hips bent—don't land with your legs straight. From here, you can immediately explode back up into the following repetition.

> **PROGRESSION:** Try to tuck your knees in at the top of the movement.

◼ JUMPING LUNGE

PREREQUISITE: Split Squat, Squat Jump

STARTING POSITION: Begin in a split squat position with your legs apart.

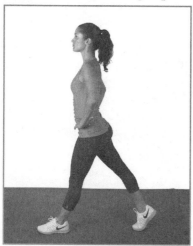

1: Initiate the movement by bending your back knee straight down. Both knees should bend the same amount and your torso should remain upright.

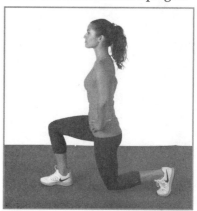

2: When you reach the bottom of the movement, drive straight up through both legs and explode into a jump. While in the air, switch your legs so that the lead leg goes to the back and the rear leg moves to the front.

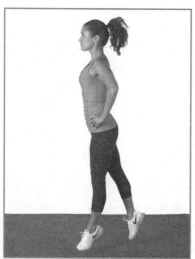

3: Land softly and back into the split squat. Both your knees should be bent as your feet touch the floor in order to absorb most of the impact of the landing. From here, you can explode back up into your next repetition.

◣ SQUAT THRUST

PREREQUISITE: Squat, Push-up, Squat Jump, Mountain Climber

STARTING POSITION: Stand upright with your feet shoulder-width apart.

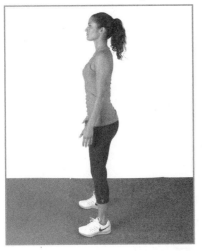

1: Squat and drop straight down, placing your hands on the floor in front of you.

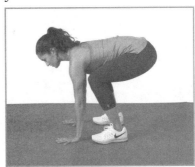

2: Shoot both legs straight back at the same time. You should end up in the top part of a push-up. Your arms and legs should be fully extended.

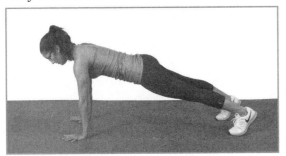

3-4: Shoot both legs back toward your hands. Then jump straight up. Land softly with your knees bent. As you land, you should continue down into the next repetition.

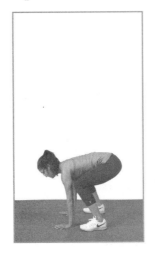
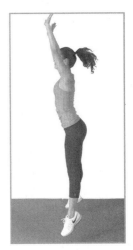

> **PROGRESSION:** Try to tuck your knees in at the top of the movement.

APPENDIX

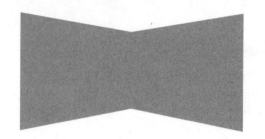

WARMING UP

It's extremely important to warm up your body before engaging in any kind of exercise. Not only does doing so get your body ready for the activity at hand, it also plays a big role in preventing injury. There are three basic ways to warm up.

A general warm-up can be any movement (such as jogging in place, jumping rope, jumping jacks) that increases the heart rate and overall blood flow throughout the body. If you have access to fitness equipment, elliptical machines, bikes and treadmills are also excellent choices. General warm-ups are especially effective prior to cardiovascular activities. Warm-ups should last 5–10 minutes and your heart rate should reach between 90–110 beats per minute (bpm). If your heart rate falls below 90, increase the intensity of your warm-up; if it exceeds 110, decrease the intensity.

Movement preparation is a method of stimulating the nervous system by targeting individual joints. This allows you to "wake up" your muscles and prepare your body for exercise. The focus of movement preparation is to mobilize the joints that rely on mobility and stabilize the joints that rely on stability. Movement preparation is a good way to warm up if you have any joint injuries or muscle imbalances. It's also good as preparation for functional and athletic movements.

Dynamic stretching is a movement-based method of stretching designed to take joints through their normal range of motion while still increasing body temperature and heart rate. Unlike static stretches, dynamic stretches are not held. This is a good way to warm up if you're preparing for movements and activities that require a large range of motion. It also helps to loosen tight or stiff muscles prior to exercise.

Time permitting, you can benefit greatly from a combination of these three types of warm-ups. Doing so will thoroughly prepare your body for exercise. If you combine the three, begin with a 5-minute general warm-up, followed by the movement preparation and then dynamic stretching.

MOVEMENT PREPARATION

FOOT CIRCLE

This improves ankle mobility. **1:** Do 10–15 complete circles in a clockwise direction and then 10–15 complete circles in a counterclockwise direction. **2:** Alternate dorsiflexion (flexing your foot) and plantarflexion (pointing your foot) 10–15 times.

SIDE LUNGE

This works on knee stability. Stand upright with both feet together, then step to your right side, bend your right knee, sit back and extend your arms forward. The other leg should be completely straight. Repeat to the other side.

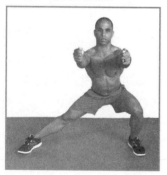

HIP MOBILITY

1: From standing, raise your right knee to hip height, keeping your thigh parallel to the floor. Maintain this position for the duration of the exercise. **2:** Fully straighten your knee and then bend it. **3:** Internally rotate your hip and then externally rotate it. **4:** Move your knee across your body and then take it out to the side.

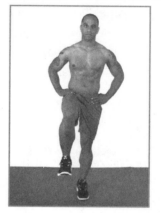

PLANK

This focuses on trunk stability. See page 161 for instructions on how to perform this exercise.

SCAPULAR PUSH-UP

This focuses on scapular (shoulder blade) mobility. **1:** From a push-up position, initiate the movement by retracting your shoulder blades together. Make sure to keep the arms straight. **2:** Extend back up by protracting your shoulders back to the starting position.

DYNAMIC STRETCHES

LUNGE ROTATE

1: From standing, step your left foot forward into a lunge. **2:** From the lunge, rotate to your left side. Repeat to the other side.

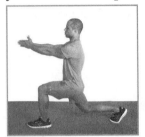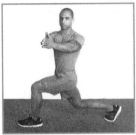

PRONE LEG ROTATION

1: Lie facedown on the floor. **2:** Bend your right knee and rotate your torso to the left until your foot touches the floor.

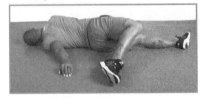

LEG SWING UP

1: Stand with both arms fully extended in front and kick one leg straight up to touch your hands. Continue alternating legs.

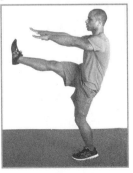

LEG SWING SIDE

1: Stand next to a wall, chair or other object for support. **2:** Swing your leg across your body as much as you comfortably can, and then swing your leg back out the side. Repeat, then switch sides.

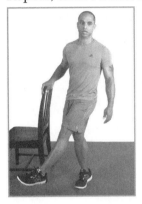

ARM SWING

1: From standing, extend one arm fully overhead and the other arm fully back behind you. **2:** Switch positions, then continue alternating.

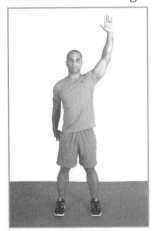

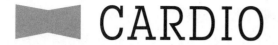 # CARDIO

In addition to resistance training, cardiovascular activity such as running, rowing, jumping rope and cycling plays a major role in increasing one's fitness level. Cardiovascular activity is any activity that uses oxygen as the body's primary source of energy. This is achieved by continuously performing submaximal movements over an extended period of time. Cardiovascular work is characterized by repetitive work at a low to moderate intensity with little to no rest.

Cardiovascular work generally has two primary functions. The first is to strengthen the heart. As our hearts get stronger, our ability to extract oxygen from our blood (VO2 max) increases. The second function is weight loss. Cardiovascular work can be designed to be sustained for as little as 10 minutes to longer than one hour. Your cardio can be completed in short and very intense intervals, or longer but moderate-intensity sessions. The higher the intensity, the less time is required.

It's important to be aware of your heart rate and/or rate of perceived exertion (RPE) when engaging in cardiovascular work. The level of intensity is inversely proportional to the amount of time you should spend. This means that if you exercise at a higher intensity, you'll require less time than exercising at a lower intensity.

TARGET HEART RATE (THR)

Your THR is the heart rate goal that you set up for cardiovascular activity. To begin, you'll have to determine your maximum heart rate (HRMax), which is the highest that your heart rate should get with exercise.

$$HRMax = 220 - age$$

For example, a 32-year-old would have a maximum heart rate of 188.

Once you have your maximum heart rate, you must then determine your intensity level.

$$60\% \; THR = HRMax \times .6$$
$$70\% \; THR = HRMax \times .7$$
$$80\% \; THR = HRMax \times .8$$

The percentage of your HRMax is directly related to the RPE scale on page 13.

STRETCHING & COOLING DOWN

Stretching can kill two birds with one stone, as it gives you the opportunity to cool down while also incorporating your flexibility training. All stretches should be held for 15–30 seconds. Move the joint to the point where you feel mild discomfort; you shouldn't be in pain. If a muscle is particularly tight, you can hold the stretch for 30 seconds, release and stretch again for another 30 seconds.

CALVES (GASTROCNEMIUS)

Facing a wall, place your hands on the wall with your arms fully extended. Split your legs so that one leg is in front and the other is extended behind you. Bend your lead leg until you feel the stretch in the rear calf. The rear heel should be on the floor with the toes pointed straight ahead; the knee should be fully extended the entire time.

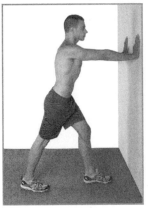

CALVES (SOLEUS)

Stand with one foot in front of the other and sit back on the heel of your rear leg. Pull the lead foot back until you feel a stretch in your calves. Make sure that the heel of your lead leg is touching the floor the entire time. To intensify the stretch, pull the lead foot back more. To make the stretch less intense, move the foot forward. Switch sides.

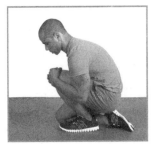

HAMSTRINGS

Stand with one foot in front of the other. Bend both knees and place both hands on the floor. Keeping your hands on the floor, straighten both legs to stretch the lead leg.

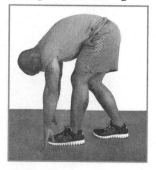

QUADS

Standing upright, bend one knee and grip your foot with the same-side hand. Pull the heel toward you with your knee pointing straight down.

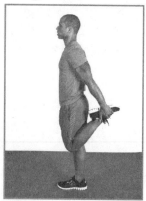

GLUTES

Lie on your back with both legs straight. Without rotating your torso, pull one knee up and across to the opposite shoulder. Switch sides.

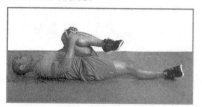

PIRIFORMIS 1

Stand with your feet together and place your left ankle on your right thigh, just above your knee. Extend your arms forward, parallel to the floor, and sit back as much as you comfortably can. Hold. Switch sides.

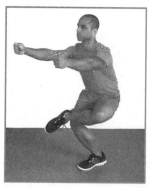

PIRIFORMIS 2

Lie on your back with both knees bent. Place your right ankle on your left thigh. With both hands, grab your left thigh and pull in. Switch sides.

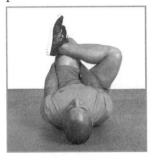

LOWER BACK

Lie on your back and pull both knees into your chest.

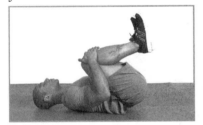

OBLIQUES

Lie on your back and lift both legs so that your hips and knees are both bent 90 degrees. Lower your knees and hips to one side until your legs touch the floor. Place your hand on the top leg and gently pull down. Extend your other arm so that both shoulders are flat on the floor. Switch sides.

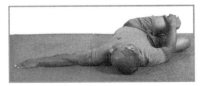

ABDOMINAL 1

Lie on your back with your arms and legs extended. Reach your arms back toward the wall behind you while simultaneously pointing your toes forward to the wall in front of you.

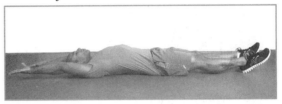

ABDOMINAL 2

Lie facedown and place your palms on the floor next to you. Press your palms into the floor, lifting your trunk off the floor.

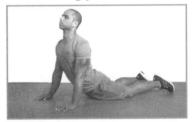

PECS

1: Stand next to a wall with your arm bent at 90 degrees and your upper arm parallel to the floor. **2:** Place your forearm against the wall. Rotate in the opposite direction while maintaining contact with the wall.

LATS

Stand underneath the doorframe pull-up bar and grip the bar with one hand. Keeping your arm straight, shoot your hips out to one side. Then shoot them out to the other side.

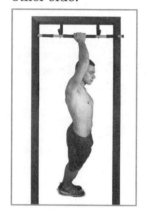

BICEPS

Stand upright with both arms at your sides and thumbs facing forward. Internally rotate your thumbs and extend your elbows as much as you can. Keeping both the rotation and the extension, reach your arms as far backward as you can.

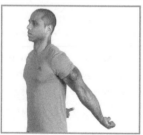

TRICEPS

Extend your right arm overhead then bend your elbow to touch the base of your neck. Use your other arm to gently pull on the elbow to intensify the stretch. Switch sides.

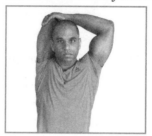

DELTOIDS

Take one arm across your chest, using your other arm to grab behind your elbow and gently pull your arm in to intensify the stretch. Switch sides.

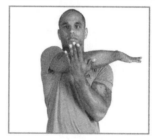

TRAPS

Bend your left arm and place it behind your back. Tilt your right ear to your right shoulder. Switch sides.

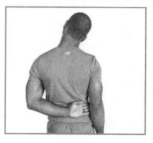

INDEX

Abdominal Curl-Up, as test, 38.
  See also Crunches
Abdominal endurance, testing, 38
Abdominal exercises, 165–68
Abdominal stretches, 191
Abdominals (abs), 9, 18
Accountability, and fitness, 22
Adductors (groin), 10
Aerobic endurance, testing, 39
Alternate-Grip Pull-Up, 99
Alternate-Grip Push-Up with Bar, 175
Alternate Single-Leg Raise, 127
Alternate Single-Leg Raise Side to Side, 128
Anaerobic endurance, testing, 39
Arm muscles, 9
Arm Swing (warm-up), 187
Assessments of fitness. *See* Fitness assessing; Fitness testing
Attitude, negative, as excuse, 24

Band-Assisted Pull-Up, 119
Bars. *See* Doorframe pull-up bars
Basal metabolic rate (BMR), 26
Baseline data, of body composition, 34–35; chart, 35
Biceps brachii, 9
Biceps stretch, 192
Bicycle Crunch, 166
Body composition, assessing, 34–35
Body measurements, 34–35
Body sculpting program (intermediate), 76–80
Boredom, as excuse, 23
Breakfast, 26, 28
Breathing, 12, 95, 159
Bridge, 150

Calf Raise, 174
Calories, 25–26, 28
Calves, 10
Calves (gastrocnemius) stretch, 189
Calves (soleus) stretch, 189
Cardio-conditioning exercises, 176–83

Cardio-conditioning programs: advanced, 85–89; intermediate, 81–84
Cardiovascular ability, 14
Cardiovascular activities, 188
Cardiovascular training, 16
Chair-Assisted Pull-Up, 118
Chair Dip, 153
Chair Squat, as test, 37–38
Chest muscles, 9
Chin-Up, 96
Close-Grip Pull-Up, 100
Coffee, 28
Concentric muscle contractions, (positive), 11
Consistency: in diet, 26–27; in programs, 42
Contractions, muscle, 11–12
"Controlled indulgence," 27
Cooling down stretching, 19, 30, 189–92
Core, 10; bracing, 12
Core Walk-Out, 172
Crunch (basic), 165
Crunches, 18, 134, 165, 166, 168; as test, 38
Curls: arm, 106; leg, 105, 123, 125, 133, 168

Daily caloric requirement (DCR), 25–26
Deltoids (shoulder), 9
Deltoids stretch, 192
Diamond Push-Up, 141
Diet, 16, 25–28; misconceptions, 28
Dip with Bar, 170
Dips, 153–54, 170
Doorframe pull-up bars, 5–7; benefits, 3–4, 6; floor exercises, 169–75
Dynamic stretches, 185, 187

Eccentric muscle contractions, (negative), 11
Efficiency, in programs, 43
Endurance, testing, 37–39
Erector spinae (lower back), 9

Excuses, 23–24
Exercise, in general, 14–16; benefits, 15; defined, 14; misconceptions, 17–19; recommendations, 15
Exercise positioning, 30
Exercises, 94–183; abdominal, 165–68; doorframe pull-up bar floor, 169–75; hanging abdominal, 122–36; lower body, 146–52; plank-based, 156, 159–64; positioning, 30; pull-ups, 94–121; push-ups, 137–45, 169, 175; terms used, 32; upper body, 153–58
Expense, as obstacle, 23
Express workouts, 92
External obliques, 9

FAQs, programs, 44–45
Fat weight, assessing, 34
Fat-free mass (FFM), assessing, 34
Fitness, 14–19; baseline data, 34–35; concepts, 42–44; defined, 14; keys to success, 20–24; misconceptions, 17–19; testing, 36–39; tracking apps/devices, 22
Fitness assessing, 34–35
Fitness testing, 36–39; abdominal curl-up, 38; chair squat, 37–38; chart, 36; plank, 39; pull-up, 36–37; push-up, 37; walk/run, 39; squat thrust, 39
Fitness goals. *See* Goals and goal setting
Fitness journal, 22
Fitness levels, assessing, 33
Fitness programs. *See* Programs
5-minute express workouts, 92
Flexibility, 16
Floor Dip, 154
Floor exercises, with bar, 169–75
Food, 16, 25–28; journal, 27; misconceptions, 28; tracking apps, 27
Foot Circle (warm-up), 186
Forearm muscles, 10

Forward Lunge, 148
Frame-Assisted Sit-Up, 173
Frustration, as excuse, 24
Full Circle, 132
Functional ability, 14
Functional training, 16

General fitness programs: beginner, 51–53; intermediate, 54–58
Girth measurements, assessing, 35
Gluteals (glutes), 9
Glutes stretch, 190
Goals and goal setting, 20–22, 33, 40–41, 46, 50; body fat, 34; chart, 41; checklist, 40; and fitness assessment/testing, 33, 34, 35, 36, 37, 38, 39; heart rate, 34; measurements, 35; weight, 34

Half Circle, 130–31
Hamstrings, 10
Hamstrings stretch, 190
Handstand Shoulder Press, 158
Hanging abdominal exercises, 122–36; technique, 122
Hanging Biceps Curl, 106
Hanging Bicycle, 135
Hanging Leg Curl, 123
Hanging Leg Curl with Rotation, 125
Hanging Oblique Crunch, 134
Hanging straps, 122
Heart problems, 29
Heart rate, 188
High Knees, 180
High Twist, 136
Hip flexors (psoas major), 9
Hip Mobility (warm-up), 186
Hydration, 16, 27, 28

Illnesses, 29; as obstacle, 23
Injuries, 29; as obstacle, 23
Intensity, of exercise, 13, 17, 18
Internal obliques, 9
Isometric Hold, 112
Isometric Hold (Side to Side), 107
Isometric muscle contractions, (static), 11

Journals: fitness, 22; food, 27
Jumping Lunge, 182

Jumping Pull-Up, 120
Jumping Pull-Up (Feet on Floor), 121

Kick-Up, 167

L-Shaped Pull-Up, 104
Lactic acid buildup, 19
Latissimus dorsi (lats), 9
Lats stretch, 192
Leg Curl, 168
Leg Curl with Extension, 133
Leg Extension, 174
Leg muscles, 9–10
Leg Swing Side (warm-up), 187
Leg Swing Up (warm-up), 187
Lifestyles: healthy, 16; sedentary, 19
Load (resistance), of exercise, 13
Lower back muscles (erector spinae), 9
Lower back stretch, 191
Lower body endurance, testing, 37–38
Lower body exercises, 146–52
Lunge Rotate (warm-up), 187
Lunges, 148, 149, 182

Macrocycles, 50
Meals, frequency, 27
Medical clearance, 23, 29
Mesocycles, 50
Milestones, 22; checklist, 40
Misconceptions: fitness, 17–19; nutrition, 28
Modified Pull-Up, 114
Modified tabata sample template, 49
Mountain Climber, 179
Movements: components, 11–12; variables, 12–13
Multivitamins, 28
Muscles, 8–10; contractions, 11–12; illustration, 8
Muscular strength, 14
Muscular strength programs: advanced, 72–75; intermediate, 68–71

Nutrition, 25–28; misconceptions, 28

Oblique Twist, 129
Obliques, 9
Obliques stretch, 191
Obstacles, to fitness, 23
1-minute squat thrusts, as test, 39
1.5 mile walk/run, 39; as test, 39
Overtraining, 44

Parallel Grip Pull-Up, 97
Partner-Assisted Pull-Up, 115
Partners, in workouts, 22
Pecs stretch, 191
Pectoralis major (chest), 9
Periodization, 44, 50
Perspiring, 17–18
Pike Press, 175
Piriformis stretches, 190, 191
Plank (basic), 161, 186; as test, 39
Plank-based exercises, 156, 159–64; breathing, 159; movement, 159; problems, 160; technique, 159; as test, 39
Plank to Side Plank, 164
Plank Walk-Up, 156
Plank with Arm Extension, 162
Plateaus, 43, 44
Posture, 29–30
Power Push-Up, 143
Press-Up, 155
Press-Up with Bar, 171
Programs, 32–92; body sculpting, 76–80; cardio conditioning, 81–89; designing, 42–44; FAQs, 44–45; and fitness assessments, 33–39; 5-minute express, 92; general fitness, 51–58; muscular strength, 68–75; pull-up development, 90–91; quick athlete's workout, 91; templates, 46–49; weight loss, 58–67
Progression, in programs, 43
Prone Leg Rotation (warm-up), 187
Protein, 28
Psoas major (hip flexors), 9
Pull-up bars. See Doorframe pull-up bars
Pull-up development program, 90–91
Pull-Up with High Leg Raise, 109
Pull-Up with Leg Curl, 105
Pull-Up with Negative Focus, 113

Pull-Up with Press-Out, 108
Pull-ups, 94–121; benefits, 6–7; breathing, 95; exercises, 96–110; preparation exercises; 7, 111–21; problems, 95; technique, 94–95; as test, 36–37
Push-Up (basic), 139; as test, 37
Push-up-based exercises, 137–45, 169, 175; movement, 138; technique, 137–38; as test, 37
Push-Up with Bar, 169
Push-Up with Rotation, 144

Quadriceps (quads), 9
Quads stretch, 190
Quick athlete's workout, 91

Range of motion (ROM), 12
Rate of perceived exertion (RPE), 13, 188
Rectus abdominis (abs), 9, 18
Repetition circuit sample template, 48
Repetitions (reps), 12, 45
Resistance training, 16
Rest/recovery, in programs, 13, 43
Resting heart rate (RHR), assessing, 34
Reverse Lunge, 149
Rewards, 22
Rhomboid major (rhomboids), 9

Scapular Pull-Up, 111
Scapular Push-Up (warm-up), 186
Sets, 12
Short-Range Pull-Up (Lower Half), 116
Short-Range Pull-Up (Upper Half), 117
Shoulder muscles, 9
Shoulder Touch, 179
Side-Facing Pull-Up, 102
Side Lunge (warm-up), 186
Side Plank, 163
Side-to-Side Pull-Up, 103

Single-Leg Bridge, 151
Single-Leg Squat, 152
Single set sample template, 46
Sit-ups, 173
Six-pack. See Abdominals
Skater, 178
Sleep, 16
Soreness, post-exercise, 17
Specificity, in programs, 42
Speed Squat, 176–77
Split Squat, 147
Sports drinks, 28
Squat (basic), 146
Squat Jump, 181
Squat Thrust, 183; as test, 39
Squat Thrust into Pull-Up, 110
Squats, 110, 146, 147, 152, 176, 181, 183
Stability, testing, 39
Staggered Push-Up, 142
Standard Pull-Up, 98
Standing Walk-Out, 157
Stomach muscles, 9, 18
Straight-Leg Raise, 124
Straight-Leg Raise Side to Side, 126
Straps, hanging, 122
Strength tests, 36, 37
Strength training, and weight loss, 19
Stress, 15; as obstacle, 23
Stretching, 19, 30, 189–92; dynamic stretches, 185, 187
Supersets sample template, 47
Sweat suits, 17–18
Sweating, 17–18

Tabata sample template, 49
Target heart rate (THR), 188
Templates (samples) for workouts, 46–49 modified tabata, 49; repetition circuit, 48; single set, 46; supersets, 47; tabata, 49; timed circuit, 48; trisets, 47
Tempo, of exercise, 12–13

Testing. See Fitness testing
Tibialis anterior (shin), 10
Time for exercise, as obstacle, 23
Timed circuit sample template, 48
Timing, of exercise, 19
"Toning up," 18
Total-Body Crunch, 168
Total-Body Explosive Push-up, 145
Tracking apps/devices: fitness, 22; food, 27
Trapezius (traps), 9
Traps stretch, 192
Triceps brachii, 9
Triceps Push-Up, 141
Triceps stretch, 192
Trisets sample template, 47

Upper back muscles, 10
Upper body endurance, testing, 37
Upper body exercises, 153–58
Upper body strength, testing, 36, 37

Vitamins, 28
VO2 max, 188; as test, 39

Walk-Outs, 157, 172
Walk/run, as test, 39
Warming up, 30, 185–87; and dynamic stretches, 185, 187; general exercises, 187; importance, 185; movement preparation, 186
Water, 16, 27, 28
Weight lifting, 18
Weight loss programs: beginner, 58–62; intermediate, 63–67
Weight loss, and strength training, 19
Weight, assessing, 34
Wide-Grip Pull-Up, 101
Wide Push-Up, 140
Women, and training, 17

ACKNOWLEDGMENTS

First and foremost, I'd like to thank my wife, Ana. She has always been an incredible source of support and inspiration, and has also very patiently put up with the chaos that is a personal trainer's schedule. I've never met a more loving and beautiful person.

There are too many friends and family to mention, but I offer thanks to my wonderful parents, Eddie and Donna, and to my closest friends, Justin, Ben, Adrian and Gary. You guys are the best friends a person could have.

Thanks to Jim and all of the staff at the McBurney YMCA, which has become a second home to me.

A huge source of knowledge and motivation has come from my teammates, Royston and the entire Guzman family for teaching me so much and helping me to develop as both an athlete and a human being.

A special thanks to all of my clients, current, past and future. It's their loyalty that has allowed me to enjoy a career that I'm passionate about.

Finally, I'm incredibly grateful to everyone at Ulysses Press for giving me this opportunity. You've been awesome to work with—thanks for the support and your confidence in me.

ABOUT THE AUTHOR

Ryan George has been a fitness professional since 2001. In that time he has gained diverse experience working with clientele from all populations, including celebrities, leaders in business, high-level professional and amateur athletes, children, post-rehab patients and many others. In addition to being a trainer, Ryan also works as an instructor for the World Instructor Training Schools, helping to develop the next generation of fitness professionals. Ryan has made appearances as a fitness expert on CBS, ABC and Livestrong.com. In 2006, Ryan founded My Home Trainer, a fitness company specializing in working with clients in their homes. Ryan currently runs his own blog and podcast that can be found online at www.RyanGeorgeFitness.com.